T5-DHE-125

JOHN P. SAVAGE
176 PORTLAND STREET
DARTMOUTH, N. S.

Contraception

CONTRACEPTION

Copyright © Canada 1971 by Harvest House Ltd.
All rights reserved.

Library of Congress Catalog Card No. 70-178727
ISBN 88772 122 2
Deposited in the Bibliothèque Nationale du Québec
4th quarter, 1971

First Harvest House edition — December 1971
For information address Harvest House Ltd.,
1364 Greene Ave., Montreal 215, Quebec, Canada.

This book was first published in the French language
by Les Editions de L'Homme, Montreal.

Printed and bound in Canada

translated by Jane Brierley

Contraception

Lionel Gendron M.D.

 Harvest House, Montreal

By the Same Author

Birth : The Story of How You Came to Be

CONTRACEPTION

"We can and do praise the book ... especially the good-humoured way it treats facts of contraception that are so important to all of us. Implicit in the whole work is the range of ways in which our sexual lives affect everything else we accomplish, and the very quality of life for individuals.

The illustrations, eschewing as they do the usual anatomical diagrams, reflect the pleasant approach; they give the reader agreeable bodies to look at, corresponding to our contemporary ideal of mature beauty.

Because of this, and because Dr. Gendron obviously understands the psychology of sex, and of living together, we'd give this book to anyone, from 11 to 12 years on for information."

K.G. MARSHALL, M.D. (McGill), FRCP (Canada), Associate, Royal Victoria Hospital, Gynecology, Associate, Professor of Pathology, McGill University

MARY MARSHALL, R.N., B.A. (McGill)

Contents

Chapter 14

Chapter 15

Chapter 16

Chapter 17

Introduction

In my eighteen years as a general practitioner and obstetrician, I have always considered the emotional and sexual life of a couple to be of the greatest importance, both during and after the child-bearing years. I wanted to free my patients (and sometimes their husbands) from their subconscious acceptance of all the taboos surrounding sex and pregnancy. I also did my best to give a clear description of the biological facts. In this way, many couples have been able to gain a more mature approach to parenthood. For me, the experience has been among the most rewarding of my career.

For a couple who is well-prepared, each three-month period during pregnancy produces new emotional and erotic feelings. A sex life in which both partners actively share gives the woman an added degree of femininity, and the man an enhanced virility. Together they attain a new range of sensations through a succession of emotional and physical experiences. The atmosphere in which they live is happy and serene, and they thus preserve the original charm and ardour of married love.

After their children were born, many couples were obliged, in years gone by, to adopt fairly limited methods of contraception. As a result, sex and family life did not combine well, and I have witnessed severe marital problems caused by unwanted pregnancies. Fortunately, several effective methods of contraception have been positively explored by modern medical researchers and clinicians, among them the hormone method. Family planning has become a reality. With medical science as its guide, society has acquired a new sense of freedom — to the benefit of the individual human being. The importance of contraceptives which promote marital harmony has been generally recognized, and society is making an effort to prepare young people for marriages which will be more rewarding and durable.

Within the last twelve years, I myself, as well as other physicians, have undertaken an intensive family-planning program designed to promote the woman's physical and mental well-being, with a view to protecting her from unexpected pregnancies which are so often the source of marital breakdown. Further, I have attempted to help couples achieve a spontaneous and satisfying sexual relationship. Time after time I have seen wives who were depressed and ridden with anxiety become happy, active, good-humoured women through the use of the contraceptive hormone pill, commonly known as "the pill."

Couples who no longer fear unwanted pregnancies find greater fulfilment in their emotional and sexual lives. They are drawn closer together, and have more to offer their children in terms of time, money, attention and love.

LIONEL GENDRON, M.D.

Chapter 1
The Female Genital Organs

The female body contains the delicate organs commonly known as the sexual or reproductive organs. Women are often uninformed as to the exact details of their anatomy, in particular the genital region.

The Vulva

The vulva includes the following anatomical formations : **labia majora** or "major lips," **labia minora** or "small lips," the **urethra,** the **vaginal entrance,** the **clitoris, Bartholin's glands,** and the **mons veneris** or mound of Venus.

The **labia majora** or "major lips" protect the other anatomical formations mentioned above. They are formed of soft tissue covered with skin and pubic hair.

The **labia minora** or "small lips" are protected by the major lips. Their tissue is firmer, and varies with each individual between one and two inches in length. It is not unusual or abnormal for them to be longer or wider than the average, and therefore

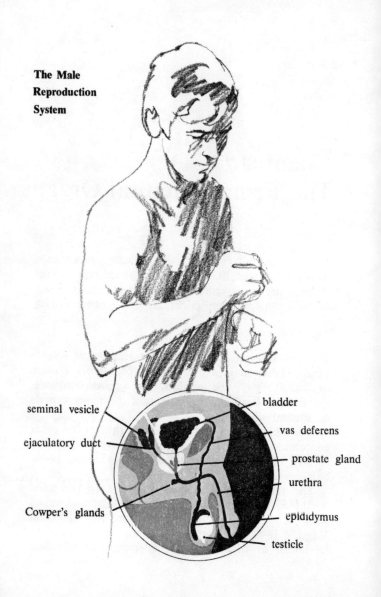

**The Male
Reproduction
System**

seminal vesicle

ejaculatory duct

Cowper's glands

bladder

vas deferens

prostate gland

urethra

epididymus

testicle

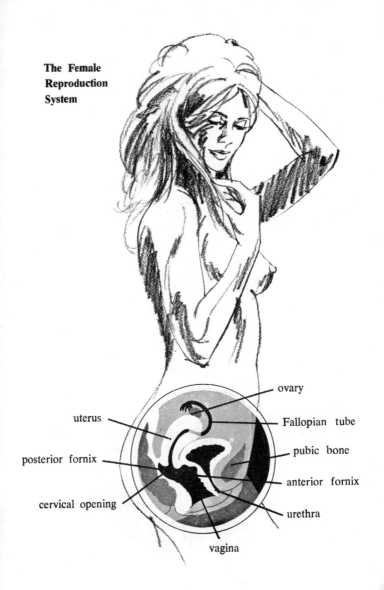

The Female Reproduction System

ovary

Fallopian tube

uterus

pubic bone

posterior fornix

anterior fornix

cervical opening

urethra

vagina

to contain more nerve endings and blood vessels. The woman whose small lips are longer has received a gift from nature, as the intensity of erotic sensitivity increases with the number of nerve endings found there.

The **urethra** is the small duct through which the bladder is emptied. The urethra opening lies above the vaginal entrance, and is in the genital area. Two glands, known as Skene's glands, are found close to the urethra. When stimulated erotically, they secrete a mucous substance which lubricates the vaginal entrance.

The **vaginal entrance** is the genital surface which extends from the clitoris to the vaginal opening. This area is highly sensitive to erotic stimulation.

The **clitoris** is a small organ capable of erection and the clitoral system is comparable to the penis in men. It is above or in front of the urethral opening. When erect, the tip of the clitoris expands to about the size of a pea, and can be easily felt. This sensitive organ seems to be the key to erotic arousal and satisfaction in most women.

The **hymen** is an elastic membrane of fairly thick fibrous tissue, found at the vaginal entrance. There is an opening in the centre, allowing the menstrual flow to pass through. It is ruptured at the time of first intercourse, usually with an accompanying loss of blood, although this is not always the case. There are many different hymens and few "ruptures," as such.

Bartholin's glands are found on either side of the vaginal entrance. When a woman is sexually aroused, these glands produce a substance which lubricates the vaginal entrance and orifice. The vagina proper is lubricated by its mucous membrane, the surface of which releases drops of serous fluid when stimulated, increasing with the heightening of erotic tension. The surface of the vagina becomes coated with this fluid. The tiny vessels in the vaginal mucous membrane are engorged with blood, and drops of serous fluid pass through a fine vascular network.

The **mons veneris** is a small cushion of adipose tissue covering the pubic symphysis — commonly referred to as the pubic bone, although it is in fact a virtually immoveable joint, with the bones connected by an elastic tissue. The mons veneris is a point of erotic stimulation, and many women receive greater satisfaction when it is delicately caressed than from the clitoris.

Ovaries and Ova (Eggs)

The female ovaries, comparable to the male testicles, are found in the abdominal cavity on either side of the uterus. At birth, a baby girl possesses millions of immature ova or eggs. In growth and maturity, they differ greatly from sperm cells. A boy at puberty is constantly producing countless sperm cells. In a girl at puberty, by contrast, one egg matures at a time, alternating between the two ovaries, within a space of twenty-eight to thirty-two days.

The **ovum** or egg is a cell with a diameter of 0.2 millimeters, four times the length of a sperm cell. It is the largest of all human cells. By examining seminal fluid under a microscope, the existence and vitality of sperm cells can be determined. This is almost impossible in the case of a human egg, as it is extremely difficult to get at. On reaching maturity, the egg is expelled from the ovary. This process is called ovulation. The exact date of this physiological phenomenon cannot be determined in advance. However, the end of ovulation can be detected by basal temperature readings, showing the rise in body temperature after ovulation.

If the egg is not fertilized, menstruation occurs between the twelfth and sixteenth day after expulsion from the ovary. The egg contains the X chromosome only, and the sex of a child will depend entirely on whether the fertilizing sperm cell contains an X or Y chromosome.

Ovarian Hormones

The ovaries secrete two types of hormone : **estrogen** and **progesterone.** Estrogen, which is secreted mainly before ovulation, stimulates growth and the mature functioning of the uterus and its glands, as well as the development of the mucous membrane (endometrium) covering the interior of the uterus. Progesterone, which is secreted after ovulation, stimulates production by the glands contained in the endometrium. During pregnancy, particularly until

Fertilization

The "privileged" sperm penetrates the egg.

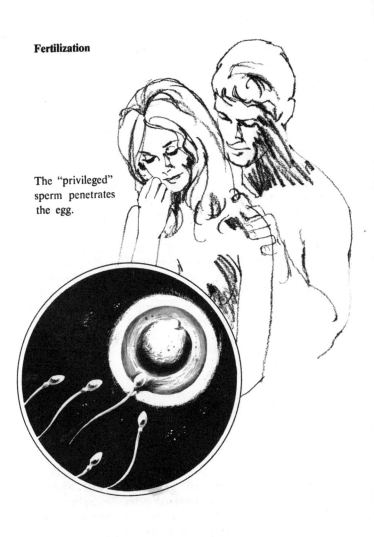

the placenta has formed, the ovaries produce a large quantity of progesterone as a natural means of preventing abortion or miscarriage.

The Fallopian Tubes and Fertilization

The two Fallopian tubes are long, narrow ducts extending from the upper end of the uterus on either side, towards the ovaries. They partially curl around the ovaries, and have fringed ends for the purpose of helping the egg pass from the ovary into the Fallopian tube. In short, they are passages between the ovaries and the uterus. As ovulation approaches, the Fallopian tube prepares to receive the egg, its fringed ends acting with a suction-like motion, somewhat resembling a sea-anemone. The egg is then pushed along the Fallopian tube towards the uterus by tiny hair-like cilia lining the interior of the tube.

The egg unites with a sperm cell. Usually fertilization takes place half-way along the Fallopian tube, which measures about twenty centimeters or seven and a half inches. The sperm cell travels on a flat surface at a speed of approximately three millimeters per minute (observed through a microscope), but takes at least eight hours to reach the area of the Fallopian tube where fertilization usually takes place.

The outside wall of the egg is covered with a sticky substance called hyaluronic acid. When this acid is dissolved by the enzyme hyaluronidase released by the sperm cell, an opening is made in the egg wall, allowing the sperm cell to penetrate. The head of the sperm cell adheres to the nucleus of the egg, which is now fertilized and continues to develop by the process of cell division.

Five days later, it enters the uterus, where a further five days are required for completing the process of nidation or implantation. The egg only remains in a condition suitable for fertilization twenty-four hours after ovulation. Once it has passed through the Fallopian tube it begins to disintegrate and can no longer be fertilized.

The Uterus

The uterus is a muscular organ, shaped like an inverted triangle, and about the size of a hen's egg. The interior is lined with a mucous membrane while the exterior is enveloped in a serous membrane. The lower end of the uterus, which leads into the vagina, is called the cervix. The uterus, ovaries and Fallopian tubes are grouped in the abdominal cavity and are protected by the pelvic bone. The uterine lining adheres to the muscular wall, and has a functional zone which responds to stimulus by the ovarian hormones (estrogen and progesterone).

This functional zone, called the endometrium, begins to develop immediately after menstruation. If a fertilized egg appears in the uterus, the endometrium welcomes and nourishes it generously. If there is no fertilized egg, the secretion of estrogen diminishes, causing the endometrium to break down and be eliminated. This is what we call menstruation. Then, once again, the cycle begins.

The Role of the Uterus in Pregnancy

The function of the uterus is to provide shelter and protection for the foetus during the nine months of pregnancy. It is hollow and pear-shaped, flexible and elastic in nature, and is contained in the pelvic cavity, in the lower abdomen. The uterus maintains a constant temperature, and is capable of stretching to accommodate the foetus without harming the other vital organs of the mother. The lower part forms the cervix, which leads into the vagina.

Each of the internal genital organs plays a vital role in the process of reproduction. Sperm cells deposited in the vagina by ejaculation swim towards the cervix, up through the uterus and into the Fallopian tubes. Here the one successful sperm cell fertilizes the egg. This is the moment of conception. If the egg is not fertilized, it passes out of the uterus unnoticed in the menstrual flow. The endometrium breaks down and is also expelled during menstruation.

The Vagina

The vagina is a cylindrical canal made of elastic tissue, leading from the vaginal opening to the uterus, and is between three and five inches in length. The front and back walls of the vagina are covered with folds which increase the erotic excitation of the penis during coitus (intercourse), and which also produce agreeable sensations in the woman. In

The Pituitary Gland
The anterior lobe of the pituitary gland regulates the stimulation of the glands generally, including the sexual glands. The pituitary is also connected in complex ways to the higher centers of the brain.

The female reproductive organs located within the pelvis.

addition, the vagina is capable of very considerable stretching, thus allowing the head of the infant to pass through during birth.

The vagina walls secrete a certain quantity of lactic acid, which increases and diminishes during the menstrual cycle. At ovulation, this vaginal secretion contains only a small quantity of lactic acid, thereby encouraging the passage of sperm cells. A highly concentrated solution of lactic acid would destroy them, but a diluted solution increases their mobility.

The vaginal wall is able to reabsorb this chemical substance by a mechanism resembling that of a suction pump, and it then passes into general circulation in the system. A whitish, clear, alkaline mucus is secreted in the cervical area, facilitating the entry of the sperm cells into the uterus at the time of ejaculation.

Chapter 2
The Male
Urogenital Organs

The male urogenital system includes : the **penis**, the **scrotum**, the **testicles** (comparable to the female ovaries), the **seminiferous tubules**, the **seminal vesicles**, and the **prostate gland.**

The Penis

The **penis** is an external organ composed of erectile tissue, the glans, and the foreskin. Normally limp, it becomes fairly rigid when an erection occurs. A canal called the **urethra** passes throughout its length from the bladder to the **meatus** or slit-like opening at the tip. The urethra has two distinct functions : the first is to empty the bladder of urine ; the second to expel the seminal fluid from the seminal glands.

The penis becomes erect if it is sexually aroused. Its dimensions and consistency then alter. When stimulation occurs, the Cowper's glands secrete a mucous substance which lubricates the urethra before the sperm is ejaculated. This physiological phenomenon resembles the lubrication of the vagina and vulva in the woman.

What exactly causes **erection**? The spongy erectile tissue forming the body of the penis becomes engorged with blood. The rigid and expanded condition thus obtained encourages satisfactory coitus (sexual intercourse). The mechanism of erection is extremely sensitive to the least disorder in the nervous system. Its activity is affected by a man's thoughts and his state of mind.

A man who is worried unconsciously sets up a reaction against erotic stimulation, and becomes incapable of erection. Psychological conflicts affect men who are sensitive, highly emotional or inexperienced in sex.

Erection is not only produced by erotic thoughts, although this is the principal reason for it, but also by a full bladder (particularly in the morning), friction of the penis, manual manipulation (masturbation), and irritation of the glans.

Apart from its urinary function, the penis plays a sexual role in procreation and the erotic satisfaction of man and woman. The glans is an erotic zone which is particularly sensitive around the base, giving agreeable sensations when touched, as well as during coitus.

The Scrotum

The scrotum is a sac of muscular tissue containing the testicles.

The Testicles

The testicles are the male sex g'ands. They are oval in shape, and are suspended in the scrotum. The left testicle is slightly lower than the right. A cross-section of this gland shows numerous seminiferous tubules fi'led with sperm cells. These are ejaculated from the penis at the moment of sexual climax. The tubules run into a common duct, called the epididymus. The vas deferens (deferent duct) transports the sperm from the epididymus to the penis.

After leaving the testicles, the sperm cells are stored in two reservoirs behind the prostate gland, called the seminal vesicles. At the moment of ejaculation, the sperm cells pass into the section of the urethra near the prostate by means of two ejaculatory ducts.

Seminal Fluid

Ejaculated seminal fluid is composed of sperm cells and secretions from the prostate, the seminal glands, and the urethra. Ejaculation is brought on by spasmodic contractions of the muscle fibres of the penis. The seminal fluid is whitish, and has a not unpleasant odour. The amount of seminal fluid ejaculated is about one tablespoon. It contains millions of sperm cells which can be seen through a microscope.

The Prostate

The prostate is a genital gland surrounded by a muscle. The g'andular section produces a liquid which forms part of the seminal fluid. The muscle contracts at the moment of ejaculation, shooting the seminal fluid into the urethra and out of the penis.

With age, this gland has an unhealthy tendency towards hypertrophy (enlargement). No one knows why. Possibly it is connected with an imbalance in production of sexual hormones. Whatever the reason, it is a clinical fact that a great many men suffer after 60 from hypertrophy of the prostate.

The location of this gland is a potential problem, as it encircles the urethra at the point where the latter enters the bladder. Increase in the size of the prostate causes pressure on the urethra, and urination becomes difficult.

The discomforts caused by this pathological condition include : difficult or frequent urinating, retention of urine, secondary infections of the bladder and kidneys, and other organic disorders.

In the majority of cases, the hypertrophy is benign. Removal of the prostate (prostatectomy) is eventually necessary in some men. Many men fear impotence as a side-effect, but there is no reason to do so, as in most cases the sexual functions are not seriously affected. The only inconvenience is retrograde ejaculation, i.e. the seminal fluid falls back into the bladder instead of being pushed out through the urethra.

Chapter 3
The Menstrual Cycle

A young girl's first menstruation ushers in a most important period of her life. This period produces changes in the adolescent girl's endocrine glands, as well as in her physique and emotional behaviour.

First Menstruation

First menstruation usually occurs between the twelfth and fourteenth year, depending on several factors. Heredity plays a considerable part, and a girl's menstrual calendar is generally similar to that of her mother and sisters. Environment, physical condition and socio-economic level also influence the date of first menstruation. Better nutrition, a psychologically favourable atmosphere and good health generally produce early and normal menstruation.

This change does not take place all at once. Change in the human organism is never sudden. The physiological process leading the young girl to physical maturity is fairly slow and steady. What are the signs ? Towards the age of ten, eleven, or twelve years, gradual changes occur. The breasts become pointed and continue to develop as the girl enters her teens. The pelvis becomes larger and fatty deposits appear on the hips. The pubic hair darkens and becomes thicker.

When menstruation occurs, this is the true sign of physical maturity in the young girl. Menstruation can be defined as the periodic shedding of the uterine lining through the vagina, during the active reproductive life of a woman. It is completely stopped by pregnancy, and in many cases during nursing of an infant. Normally, menstruation occurs regularly every twenty-eight to thirty-two days, from puberty until menopause. The menstrual flow usually lasts about five days. The amount of blood flow varies : it increases during the first day, is greatest during the second and third days, decreases the fourth day, and stops the fifth or sixth day.

At about fourteen or fifteen years, the ovaries begin to produce eggs. The girl then becomes a real woman, since she can conceive children. Some adolescent girls attain their maximum physical development at sixteen or seventeen, others between eighteen and twenty, depending on heredity and hormone activity.

Changes in the Genital Area

The mons veneris, or fatty cushion over the pubic bone, becomes more apparent. The labia majora or "major lips" become thicker, thus hiding the rest of the vulva. The labia minora or "small lips" become fuller, and the Bartholin's glands grow larger in preparation for the secretion of vaginal fluid needed during intercourse. The vascular system of the clitoris also develops, thus making erection possible. The vagina deepens in colour ; its lining thickens and becomes more resistant to coital irritation. The vaginal secretions increase in acidity. The uterus grows year by year, reaching normal size at about eighteen years. The ovaries begin secreting sexual hormones at about fifteen or sixteen years. The breasts develop fairly slowly, depending on hormone balance and heredity.

The Menstrual Process

In order for menstruation to occur normally, certain sections of the brain must be sufficiently developed. These sections are : the hypothalamus (governing emotional behaviour) ; and the antehypophysis (anterior lobe of the pituitary gland). In addition, the ovaries must be physiologically normal. At eleven years, the antehypophysis, stimulated by the hypothalamus, secretes hormones known as the gonadotrophins, which act on the gonads, i.e. the ovaries. The hormones in question are : the follicle stimulating hormone (FSH), and the luteinizing hormone (LH).

At about the same age, somatotrophine (a hormone stimulating body growth), the thyrotrophic hormone (which stimulates the thyroid gland), and corticotrophin (which controls the activity of the adrenal cortex),

Menstruation
1st to 5th day

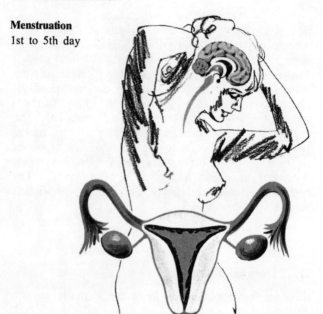

are secreted in greater quantities by the antehypophysis. They accelerate skeletal and muscular development and complete the process of maturation: that is the process leading to the complete development of the thyroid and adrenal glands.

Stimulated by the pituitary hormones, the ovaries become more oval in shape and the follicles begin to develop more markedly. The follicle is a small sac containing an ovocyte or young egg which will

FSH, First Hormone in the Menstrual Cycle

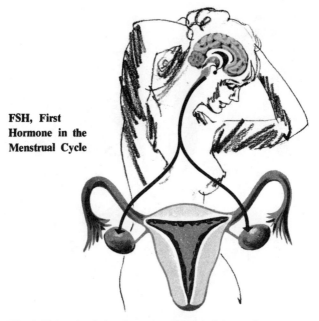

The follicle stimulating hormone (FSH) originates in the pituitary gland (hypophysis). It stimulates the ovaries, which secrete estrogen.

be expelled at ovulation, when the Graafian follicle is fully developed.

The endometrium (the mucous lining of the uterus) and the endometrial glands develop as puberty approaches. When the uterus and ovaries are sufficiently mature, first menstruation occurs. In general, a girl's first period is anovular, meaning that it is not preceded by ovulation, which may be delayed

6th to 13th day
LH (luteinizing
hormone) stimulates
development and
expulsion of egg.

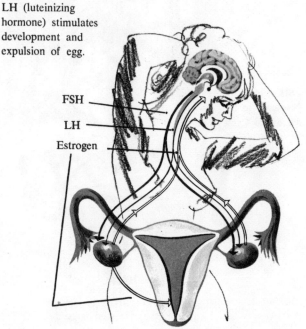

FSH

LH

Estrogen

for several months or even longer after first menstruation. The first period is brought on by a decrease in estrogen, which causes the endometrium to
break down and come away from the uterus. Ovulation
depends on how mature the ovaries are, and on
production by the pituitary glands of the two hormones: LH (the luteinizing hormone which stimulates development of the egg, ovulation, and the
formation of the corpus luteum — a yellow endocrine

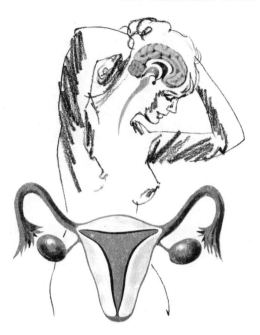

Estrogen prepares the endometrium (mucous uterine lining) for nidation of the egg.

body which is a hormone-secreting gland); and luteotrophin, which also stimulates the corpus luteum. The luteinizing hormone and luteotrophin stimulate the formation of the corpus luteum, which manufactures progesterone. This substance plays a part in breast development, the regular onset of menstruation and, if the egg is fertilized, contributes to various aspects of pregnancy.

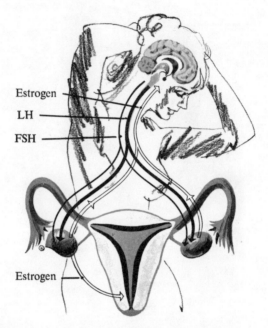

Ovulation occurs when LH (luteinizing hormone) activity is greatest (LH is the third hormone in the cycle).

Hormonal Interaction of the Pituitary and Ovaries

The menstrual cycle is normally governed by the rhythmical activity of the pituitary and ovaries. Initially, the pituitary gonadotrophins stimulate the secretion of estrogen, and after ovulation, the development of the corpus luteum which in turn secretes

Ovulation

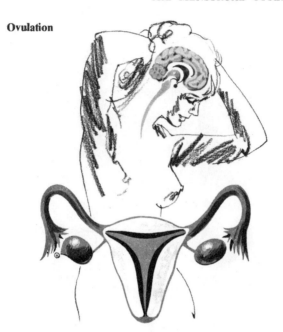

progesterone. The excess production of estrogen stops the gonadotrophin secretion. This cannot occur, however, if the anterior lobe of the pituitary is being stimulated by a small quantity of estrogen.

Physiologically, the pituitary and the ovaries form an inseparable complex. Progesterone does not seem to act directly on the gonadotrophic pituitary. Lutein only appears to affect the pituitary in the form of folliculino-luteinic deposits.

15th to 21st day

2nd stage of the
cycle. Progesterone
(4th hormone in
the cycle.)

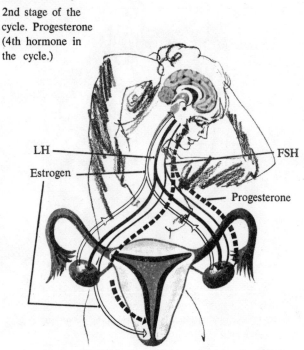

LH

FSH

Estrogen

Progesterone

Folliculine and lutein must operate simultaneously if the endometrium is to develop. Excess amounts of folliculine prevent the formation of the corpus luteum and therefore inhibit lutein secretion. The pituitary gland ceases its activity, and as a result does not produce the luteinizing hormone (LH). On the other hand, an excess of lutein encourages the elimination of folliculine. A lack of sufficient

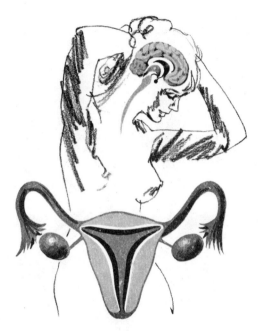

The endometrium or mucous uterine lining develops
when stimulated by progesterone.

folliculine could thus occur, resulting in insufficient
pituitary activity through lack of stimulation.

Menstruation is not merely the passage of blood
from the uterus through the vagina. The whole body
is affected. Various changes take place during the
cycle, affecting the nervous system and emotional
behaviour. From the beginning to the middle of
the cycle, body temperature is somewhat lower. It

22nd to 28th day

Signal to pituitary to withold LH. Menstruation approaches.

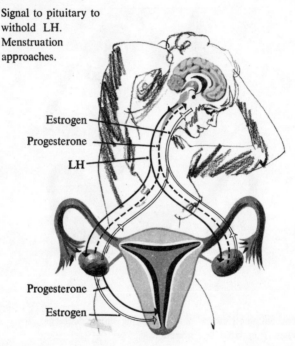

Estrogen

Progesterone

LH

Progesterone

Estrogen

rises during ovulation and then falls gradually until menstruation.

Physical change also takes place through increased retention of water in the body tissues. This is why many women complain of swelling in the second half of their cycle.

These physiological changes appear to affect the nervous system and emotional behaviour. Women

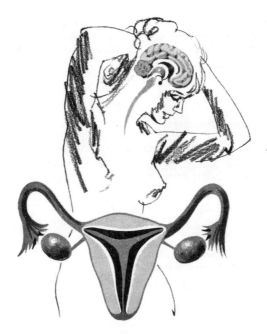

The endometrium has reached maximum development.

are generally more irritable and easily upset during the second half of the menstrual cycle. Taken all together, the physiological changes are the source of pre-menstrual tension, although this varies from one individual to another.

A woman often experiences a feeling of release when her menstrual period begins. Body temperature drops, extra water in the tissues gradually disperses, and her nervous and emotional condition improves. At this time a woman is good-humoured, less prone to irritation, more understanding and less likely to worry needlessly.

Menstrual Disorders

The first menstrual period may be early or late, with little discharge or an excessive amount, and perhaps accompanied by pain. Dysmenorrhoea — premenstrual or menstrual discomfort or pain — is unusual during the first two years of puberty, since such symptoms are nearly always connected to the ovarian cycle.

The absence in the anovular cycle of a progesterone-producing phase, which would inhibit FSH production, causes the ovaries to produce excessive quantities of estrogen. The endometrium is thus subject to continual stimulation, giving rise to functional bleeding.

Menstruation is considered late if it does not take place by the age of sixteen. By eighteen, absence of menstruation can be classified as amenorrhoea. The cause can be physiological, anatomical, psychological or constitutional. It might be hypothyroidism (deficiency of thyroid hormone), obesity, the absence of uterus and vagina, an infection, bad health, adrenal lesion or mental disorder due to environmental causes.

Early menstruation, (before the age of nine), accompanied by secondary sexual characteristics (such as growth of pubic hair, etc.), may be idiopathic, meaning of spontaneous origin, constitutional, or due to some organic disease. Ovarian tumours or cysts sometimes cause early menstruation.

Adrenal tumours often cause the appearance of masculine traits, and bring on puberty. In its idiopathic or constitutional form, early menstruation is accompanied by a complete ovarian cycle. Estrogen and progesterone are secreted, and a mature egg develops regularly. Pregnancy is therefore possible.

From the biological descriptions which I have given in this chapter, the reader will realize that the menstrual cycle is subject to various physical, physiological, endocrine and psychological influences.

Chapter 4
A New Human Science

This book is specially geared to the needs of the married couple. I have therefore attempted to make it a study of family planning through contraception, so that couples may have a true understanding of the meaning of conception. It should enable them to accept the new baby and their parental role more readily, because they have chosen when to have a child. With family planning and effective contraception, a couple can lead a happier, more tranquil life, instead of living in constant anxiety and fear of unwanted pregnancy.

This new human science — family planning combined with contraception — was the product of past errors. Did our forbears who had their usual dozen children do so with a full understanding of the miracle and responsibility of conception? Or were their families large simply because fear of social and religious taboos made family planning well-nigh unthinkable?

Family planning is the search for balance and harmony between marriage-partners. Overwhelming responsibility almost always creates severe mental and emotional stress as well as contributing to marriage breakdown, especially in modern times when a large family finds life complicated and difficult.

Family planning means bringing into the world children who are wanted and waited for with loving expectation. Conception is the great miracle of nature. Almost as wonderful is the period of waiting — pregnancy — while the infant slowly develops in his mother's womb. Because the child is desired and conceived in a spirit of mutual love, his coming brings great joy to his parents. He will grow up in a home where this spirit of mutual love can prosper, where the demands of rearing numerous children are not so overwhelming as to crush it.

The History of Contraception

For centuries, man has been looking for a contraceptive that is one hundred per cent effective. The early Egyptians used vaginal suppositories made of gum arabic. The lactic acid contained in it probably inhibited the activity of sperm cells. The ancient Greek philosopher Aristotle believed in limiting the human population by abortion. Greek writers of this period speak of the use of oil mixed with various substances and inserted in the vagina as a contraceptive. The oil hinders the progress of sperm cells through the uterus.

The Chinese favoured abortion, but their proscriptions were toxic, containing enough lead to cause poisoning. More recently, Japanese prostitutes used an oiled paper disc to cover the cervix. The Mahommedans used various chemical pessaries (vaginal suppositories). If pregnancy occurred, a probe was inserted into the uterus, which was likely to cause severe infection.

In later times, Casanova mentions the use of a gold ball inserted in the vagina before intercourse, which he claims was totally effective in preventing conception. Another mechanical device is the condom — a prophylactic sheath covering the penis. The great anatomist Fallope, who was the first to describe the Fallopian tubes which are named after him, is said to have developed the first condom. It had been in use for centuries, however, possibly as far back in time as Ancient Rome. In modern times it has been used as a preventative for venereal disease. Initially, the condom was quite short and made of linen. Later it became longer, and animal gut was used. Now, vulcanized rubber and latex have provided more adaptable materials for the condom.

Another mechanical method of contraception is the use of an occlusive cap over the cervix, commonly referred to as a diaphragm. Dr. Edward Bliss Foote is considered to have invented it. The diaphragm prevents the sperm cells from entering the uterus. In addition, a spermaticide is applied to the diaphragm before intercourse. When it first appeared, the diaphragm was made of vulcanized rubber, and later of plastic and latex.

In 1920, a German doctor by the name of Gräfenberg theorized that the presence of a foreign body in the uterus would inhibit conception. A silver ring was used, but this method was dropped, as the silver caused infection. Lately, however, developments in the plastic industry have solved this problem, and intra-uterine devices (IUD) are frequently employed.

A Leap Forward in the Science of Contraception

In 1955 an American endocrinologist, Dr. Gregory Pincus, discovered that it was possible to control the activity of female hormones and therefore to prevent conception. He carried out experiments which were successful, and his method of oral contraception was proved — thanks to the co-operation of many women who volunteered to use it. Later, he completed his clinical tests in Puerto Rico and Haiti. Today, the oral contraceptive method is very nearly perfect, and in a few years will be completely so.

Before going into detail about the hormone pill, let us briefly consider other possible methods of effective contraception. For example, would sterilization not be the best and most convenient solution for both men and women? Surgical section of the seminal ducts in men and the Fallopian tubes in women can prevent conception, but the process is virtually irreversible.

What about totally effective contraception in the form of vaccination, where the wife is "vaccinated" against her husband's sperm cells? Perhaps. The sperm cells would be immobilized before reaching the egg. Men could be sterilized in a similar way, thereby halting sperm production.

The IUD is a convenient form of temporary sterilization. This method entails the insertion of a small piece of plastic in the uterus by a gynecologist.

From the standpoint of administering contraceptives, the best method would seem to be a pill taken by mouth — a long-acting pill would be an ideal solution — or a simple injection, if a suitable substance could be perfected.

The Low-dose Pill

Some women fear that the low-dose pill will not give them perfect protection. They are wrong. Oral contraceptives have been developed to the maximum degree of security. The compounds used in preventing ovulation have now been reduced to a very small dose. Included in the low-dose pill are small amounts of estrogen and the substances involved in the second phase of endometrial growth.

The total hormone content administered orally is about one milligram. Side-effects are minimized, and a great many more women are able to use this low-dose pill — to the benefit of their physical and mental well-being. *

Is the pill one hundred per cent effective ? Yes, if it is properly used. The woman begins hormonal

* The pill as all other modern means of contraception has its critics. I have not ignored competent studies and valid evidence about adverse reactions to the pill, nor am I unaware of the even greater research effort that is being applied to its improvement. I have chosen not to explore the issue in either direction at length here. But the concerned reader should make a point of discussing such matters with his, or her, physician.

contraceptive treatment five days after the beginning of menstruation. *Not the sixth day.* Even if small flecks of blood appear during the treatment, she must continue to take the pills. If menstruation occurs before the end of the treatment, she starts taking the pills again eight days after having taken the last pill in the preceding treatment.

To simplify, the best means of being protected is always to resume treatment eight days after the last pill. In effect, if your last pill was taken Sunday, resume treatment on Monday week. In this way there will be no surprise pregnancies.

The effectiveness of the contraceptive pill containing a very low dose of combined hormones has yet to be surpassed. Women who are afraid of becoming pregnant will tell me they are highly skeptical. Yet the pill offers a sure method of contraception and a release from anxiety.

The pill operates in three ways. First, it inhibits ovulation. But even if, for some unknown reason, ovulation did take place, there is a second barrier to pregnancy : the pill stimulates production by the cervix of a mucus which is hostile to sperm cells. As the sperm must pass through the tiny opening of the cervix to reach the egg, this hostile mucus acts as a strong deterrent. However, should there be sperm cells which are so resistant and powerful as to pass through this cervical barrier, there will still be no pregnancy, even if fertilization has occurred. This is because, as a third precaution, the pill speeds up changes in the endometrium, thus preventing the egg from finding suitable shelter and nourishment. In short, nidation will not take place, and an unwanted pregnancy will not occur. The absolute protection of the pill has been proved by millions of women in the course of research.

Family Planning

Family planning is the subject of much discussion today. As an example, let us take a young couple of eighteen or nineteen, who fell in love a bit too soon. The young husband and wife simply do not have the maturity to encounter daily problems without becoming depressed and despondent. The least difficulty discourages them, and they are easily beaten.

Reality is a hard and often cruel awakening for young, unprepared newly-weds. Many of these couples become parents during the first year of marriage. They have hardly had time to become used to one another before they are forced to share their love and affection with their child. All too often, they are incapable of accepting it without rebelling. The poor baby of such immature parents is in for a hard time.

Statistics prove that a large percentage of young marriages happen because of premarital pregnancy. At least fifty per cent of young couples would not have married if they had not been forced to do so for this reason. It's a disastrous beginning for any household, and ignorance of the means of contraception is the cause.

It cannot be repeated often enough : adequate sex education is of prime importance. If they were better informed, young people would be able to understand the meaning of love as a basis for their life together, and to appreciate sex as a part and not the whole substance of a relationship between two human beings.

A Perfect Hormonal Combination

The combination of hormones in the contraceptive pill not only ensures contraception; it also solves the problem of menstrual irregularity, lessens the effects of menopause, and enables women better to enjoy middle age.

I know a wife and mother of thirty-two: good-humoured, active and happy. She takes the pill. She and her husband enjoy life; they find amusement and relaxation in the company of their three children. It is an ideal family group. The wife's gay and serene expression reflects her sense of well-being. Hers is not the expression of a woman preoccupied and depressed by fears of another pregnancy. She looks radiant, has no worries about unwanted pregnancies and finds fulfilment in her emotional and sexual life.

By contrast, consider another woman, discouraged by an unwanted pregnancy and considering abortion. She claimed that she did not want any more children, having two already and feeling she couldn't handle more. However, after serious consideration, she decided to go through with the pregnancy. Her mental and physical state during this period was pitiful. She suffered from nausea and uncontrollable vomiting; she complained of discomfort in various parts of her body, including lumbar pains and, in particular, congestion in the genital area. What is more, she absolutely refused to have intercourse in order to *punish* her husband for his imprudence. This was a flat rejection of marital sex, and almost nothing could save this woman's marriage.

The problem arose because Mrs. X had miscalculated. Her periods had been irregular for the past few months, and she hadn't paid attention. She should have consulted her doctor in order to have her menstrual cycle regulated. Here is a woman who did not want any more children, who was having irregular periods — and yet she waited until she became pregnant to do something about it. By then there was nothing to be done but wait out the pregnancy.

Menstrual Regularity and Hormone Balance

After ovulation, the corpus luteum forms in the ovary and secretes the hormone progesterone, in expectation of the fertilization and nidation of the egg. If the egg is not fertilized, menstruation occurs normally and regularly in the majority of women. Without ovulation, progesterone is not secreted. Menstruation is then irregular and often excessive.

Progesterone is therefore essential to good hormone balance and to a regular menstrual cycle. In addition, it protects the lining of the uterus from disease. Progesterone also has a stabilizing effect on mental and physical health, and is not merely a factor in the reproductive process. Menstrual irregularity should be treated by administration of a balanced combination of hormones.

Conception Between Forty and Fifty

Conception at this age is rare, but still possible. For her own physical and mental well-being, a woman should protect herself from an unwanted pregnancy which could be a source of marital breakdown. To have a false sense of security is always unhealthy. Modern medicine enables women to have a spontaneous sex life without fear of pregnancy, through the use of the estrogen-progesterone combination. (This treatment will one day be available to all women, including those in the lower income bracket — if it is not already, as it should be.)

Once over forty, a woman who becomes pregnant often suffers an emotional shock. The doctor makes a point of giving his older patients the information necessary for their physical and mental protection. With medical supervision, such pregnancies as do occur at this age are generally normal.

However, it cannot be denied that with late pregnancies there is a risk of pathological abortion, premature birth, prolonged labour, Caesarian section, cardio-vascular ailments and mental trouble. As far as the child is concerned, there is a risk of congenital malformation and mental deficiency. Nevertheless, one must not overstate the case : many women who become pregnant after forty have a happy ending to their pregnancy.

Menopause

Menopause is the gradual exhaustion of the ovaries. Fairly marked changes in endocrine balance take place during this long period. In many women, a drop in glandular activity begins during their thirties. The combination of estrogen and progesterone found in the contraceptive pill conserves hormone balance during menopause. It seems to me that once ovulation has ceased, the pill is a completely effective treatment for menopause, since the two female hormones are present.

Modern medicine has made great progress. Its methods make possible a longer life span, and hormone research has provided the possibility for women of a prolonged youthfulness, which should make for a happy old age — if indeed "old age" is not a term to be eliminated from our vocabulary. Towards forty-five, a woman loses some of her ovarian hormones; after fifty she loses almost all. She then needs hormone replacement therapy, which I personally consider the miracle of our modern age.

Chapter 5
The Ogino-Knaus Method

The rhythm method, more accurately known as the "Ogino-Knaus method," is based on the fact that each woman ovulates at a specific time during her menstrual cycle.

For women whose cycle is perfectly regular, this method might be reliable. It is applied as follows: in the case of a twenty-eight-day or thirty-day cycle, intercourse is avoided between the ninth and nineteenth day, i.e. the period during which the egg can be fertilized.

Conception is possible only during the short period in the menstrual cycle when ovulation takes place, that is, when the right or left ovary releases an egg. The egg remains fertilizable, for at least forty-eight hours. Ovulation can take place on almost any day of the menstrual cycle, but it usually occurs about the fourteenth day after the beginning of menstruation.

The rhythm method at one time had a great many followers; it also produced a great many babies.

It was adopted most readily by members of religions which did not countenance contraception except by total abstinence. This method eliminates sexual relations at the very moment when a woman is most inclined to have them, with a resulting frustration and discouragement of sexual desire.

Generally speaking, the rhythm method is not reliable. Women whose cycles are absolutely regular — I would say almost to the hour — can use it effectively, but they are rare. Even then, ovulation can be late, and fertilization can result.

The demands of love and the calendar are not always compatible. Young couples who submit themselves to the constraint of the rhythm method often complain later of difficulty in adapting to married life. The cause does not appear to be lack of love or inability to control their sexual urges. Rather, their capacity for erotic spontaneity has been damaged.

During the first two or three years of marriage, some couples find this method quite suitable, as they are not opposed to possible pregnancy. However, once one or two children have appeared on the scene, the couple begins to worry. The rhythm method is no longer helpful to their physical and emotional balance, and their attraction for each other tends to diminish and lose its charm. Even the most ardent love cools with years of marriage if the emotional and sexual relationship is not kept alive. Many couples who very much want to live happily together for the rest of their lives experience this. In the long run, the rhythm method becomes a source of frustration.

Menstrual Cycle
Period of Greatest Fertility (grey area)

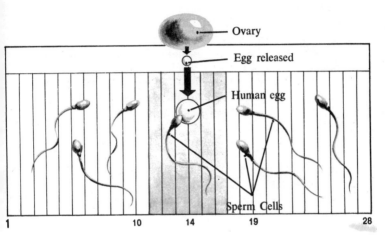

Conception only occurs during the short period after expulsion of an egg by the right or left ovary.

Sex and family life go well together in early married life. Later, husband and wife often become immersed in the monotony of daily life, leaving aside the romantic and sentimental feeling which enlivens a happy home.

This feeling disappears altogether if it is not maintained or replaced by a profound and genuine emotional tie between husband and wife. If the rhythm method is responsible for such cooling of affection between husband and wife, they should adopt an absolutely sure method of contraception in order to recreate feelings of love and tenderness as well as erotic interest.

The rhythm method suits some women who are not very fertile. However, those who are normally fertile can expect to become pregnant sooner or later.

Since the rhythm method has such serious drawbacks, how can a couple arrange their sexual life in order to avoid frequent pregnancies which, in the long run, will damage the wife's physical and mental health? How is it possible to maintain a spontaneous sex life without running the risk of annual pregnancies, as in the days of our fathers and grandfathers?

In our day, the answer is simple. The wife (or the husband) uses a totally effective contraceptive recommended after gynecological examination. It may be the contraceptive hormone pill, the IUD (intra-uterine device); or even the condom. In any case, the physician will prescribe the one most suited to the individual situation.

Chapter 6
Basal Temperature

Basal temperature refers to the lowest temperature registered in a healthy human body. This temperature is taken in the morning on waking, and varies according to one's emotional state, physical and intellectual work, digestion, athletic activity, etc. In general, body temperature is highest at the end of the day, and a night's sleep brings it down to its lowest level again. When the temperature is taken every morning and entered on a basal temperature chart, the time of ovulation can be determined.

Ovulation is a physiological process whereby the ovary releases an egg, which then passes into the Fallopian tube to await fertilization. If this does not occur within twenty-four hours, the egg degenerates. Ovulation only takes place once in each menstrual cycle — with a few rare exceptions — about fourteen days before the next menstrual period.

Since ovulation varies with each individual, every woman must discover her own fertile period by entering her basal temperature reading throughout a whole cycle on a chart or graph which is usually given with the purchase of a thermometer. A woman's body temperature drops slightly just before ovulation, and rises a few tenths of a degree during the following thirty-six hours. The period of fertility follows this rise in temperature. This method serves as a guide to the married woman who wishes to plan her pregnancies. To be successful, the temperature readings must be exact, in which case the fertile period can be fixed with almost complete certainty.

More specifically, the sequence of temperature readings is as follows. On the first day of menstruation, the woman marks an X in the first square of her chart, but does not take her temperature. She continues until menstruation has stopped, and then begins taking her temperature each morning on waking. It is a good idea not to get up, eat, smoke or drink before taking the temperature. Shake down the thermometer the night before, in order to avoid this effort in the morning. When taking the temperature, keep the thermometer in place a full five minutes, take an exact reading, and enter the figure on the chart.

Watch carefully for the temperature drop in the middle of the cycle, and the subsequent rise. This is the time either for fertilization, if a child is desired, or for abstinence during the four or preferably five days following. If ovulation does not always occur on the same day in every cycle, there will be fewer sterile days. This method is workable, but often results in physical and mental frustration due to the infrequency of sexual intercourse.

Basal Temperature

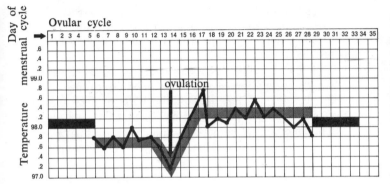

Basal Temperature

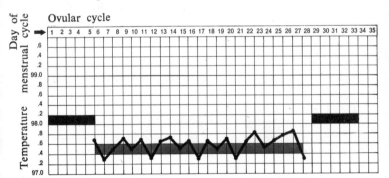

In order to determine your period of ovulation with exactitude, a basal chart should be kept for at least six consecutive months. This is an absolute necessity if the method is to be an effective contraceptive. It will only work if used with the greatest possible precision.

The doctor will help you interpret such charts when preparing for marriage or later, according to your decision. Thus he will be able to fix your fertile and sterile periods fairly accurately.

This method is sometimes suitable if a married couple have limited sexual potential and infrequent intercourse. In such a case they will be satisfied with a limited period of about ten days per month in which to have intercourse, rather than engaging in spontaneous sexual relations. However, experience has shown that frustrated men and women are usually the outcome of this method, to say nothing of anxiety, depression and unwanted pregnancies.

To realize the negative aspects of this method, one need only review past cases, before the widespread use of the hormone pill and mechanical contraceptives such as the condom, diaphragm, IUD, and spermicidal cream. Physicians' files are full of case histories of psychosomatic illness (where physical symptoms are due to emotional or mental factors) caused by sexual frustration. That conjugal morality which explicitly condemned the use of mechanical contraceptive devices (condom and diaphragm), the only means then available, proved too demanding for most couples.

Many young couples use the basal temperature method in early marriage without feeling frustrated or constrained, since they are mutually agreed on this subject. Even if they miscalculate they are not unduly upset, as they eventually want a child in any case. However, after the first pregnancy, they often decide to consult a physician about the contraceptive pill, which they would like to use for perhaps two or three years, depending on their personal decision. I should emphasize that this is entirely the business of the couple involved, and not of their respective families. Later, if they both agree to have another child, they can stop using the pill.

The choice of contraceptive can change from time to time during the active sex life of a couple. For example, they may choose the pill if they do not want further children, or the IUD if the pill is not well-tolerated.

Chapter 7
Coitus Interruptus

Coitus interruptus is the Latin term for sexual intercourse in which the penis is withdrawn from the vagina before ejaculation. Prolonged use of this method has a disturbing effect on the normal sexual mechanism of both man and woman, since it interrupts both genital and psychological contact at a critical moment.

Many men, however, use this contraceptive method regularly; and many couples become frustrated and tense after having submitted themselves to coitus interruptus for months or even years. It is then that they consult a physician in order to alter their contraceptive technique. The frustration factor involved disturbs normal sexual desires and can even destroy such desire after several years of this brusque and unfulfilling method.

On the purely physical plane, coitus interruptus is often the cause of definite uro-genital disorders, as well as a decrease in sexual ability. For women, frigidity frequently results.

Far too many women rely on this method. An inexperienced young man cannot easily control the ejaculation reflex. In any case, coitus interruptus is not an absolutely sure means of contraception. Some sperm cells may be present in the precoital fluid which flows from the penis into the vagina before actual ejaculation.

A large number of men who practise coitus interruptus just before the height of erotic excitation, and who therefore ejaculate outside of the vagina, have developed prostatitis (inflammation of the prostate gland) and vesiculitis (inflammation of the seminal vesicles) which become chronic conditions.

However, some men suffer no physical or psychological side-effects from coitus interruptus practised over a period of years. Others react severely, both physically and emotionally. It is probably safe to say that there is a fairly close link between chronic inflammation of the prostate and seminal glands, and the unhealthy mental reaction involved. The severity of the reaction varies with the individual. Some men may even become sexually neurotic; they develop a nervous condition accompanied by fear, anxiety, frustration and continual disappointment.

I would also like to say something about coitus interruptus and frigidity in women, and offer some solutions. Over the past few years, many wives have consulted me on the problem of frigidity, hoping to find the cause and the solution. In many cases the main cause was the practice of coitus interruptus used by the husband over periods of between five and fifteen years or more. It had led to sexual disappointment in the wife, who was unable to attain orgasm during intercourse.

In such cases, the doctor and his patient discuss various methods of contraception, choosing the one which is least likely to diminish erotic tension.

For example, it is not easy to stop, once sexually aroused, in order to apply diaphragm or condom. Therefore it is a good idea for women to insert a diaphragm every night and thus to be ready for intercourse. If a husband prefers to use a condom, perhaps because he feels more secure, it is preferable for him to give it to his wife before beginning to make love. She can adjust it herself when she is ready and desirous of vaginal penetration.

An Important Point

It would seem, however, that mechanical devices such as the diaphragm and condom diminish sexual pleasure. Many men and women have complained that they were less satisfied after using them. In addition, any method requiring preparation just before the beginning of intercourse is not as ideal as one which in no way reduces erotic tension. The hormone pill offers a means of contraception which does not require special preparation, and therefore does not impede the spontaneity of love-making.

For most women whose cerebro-genital response to sex is unsatisfactory because of coitus interruptus, excellent results have been obtained after the low-dose hormone pill was prescribed, according to clinical records. Freed from fear of pregnancy, more relaxed, more intent on the act of love in which they participate with mind and body, these women have been able to achieve profoundly satisfying orgasm, thus reaching the peak of conjugal erotic bliss.

Many couples have a spontaneous and satisfying sex life for a few years, particularly the child-bearing years. Between pregnancies they make do with coitus interruptus. However, once they no longer wish to have more children, they begin to suffer from nervous tension and almost morbid fear of pregnancy. Often the wife is subject to menstrual irregularity. Ideally, such a couple would, by mutual consent, consult a physician in order to obtain the most adequate form of contraceptive, particularly with reference to the wife's physical and emotional state. Their aim is to improve their sex relations, as a foundation for a continuing happy married life.

Long-standing use of coitus interruptus has, as I have said, an unhealthy effect on the physical and emotional state of the couple. I won't say that it actually destroys their health, but it does prevent them from achieving complete relaxation. The sexually frustrated or unsatisfied man or woman may develop psychosomatic symptoms, usually in the pelvic region.

There is no doubt that part of married happiness depends on sexual fulfilment. Good spirits and joy in living go hand-in-hand with such fulfilment. One's personality develops and is enriched more easily in an atmosphere of physical and mental contentment.

The beneficial aspects of a consummated sex act are denied the man and woman who practise coitus interruptus. Among the most important of these aspects are the prolonged caresses during the final phase of the erotic cycle — that is, the phase of vascular decongestion, muscle release, and cerebral ecstasy.

As the years pass, tension caused by repeated interruption of the act of love builds up, and marital harmony is disrupted. With most such couples, the wife suffers from menstrual irregularity and the hormone pill is therefore prescribed. It promotes improved hormone balance, regulates menstruation, inhibits ovulation, prevents fertilization and pregnancy.

An equally unfortunate result of reliance on coitus interruptus is typified in the case of a young woman who consults a physician, somewhat embarrassed at having to announce her pregnancy. She is a medical student, and is therefore aware of the different methods of contraception. How, then, can we account for her predicament ? One fine evening she completely forgets her theoretical studies of sperm cells and ova, and trusts to her boyfriend, who claims to be able to control ejaculation perfectly. He persuades her that coitus interruptus is a foolproof method of contraception.

What a mistake ! There is always the possibility of sperm cells being present in the precoital fluid, and interrupting intercourse before ejaculation is not a sure form of protection. The couple only need make love once to bring about pregnancy, if that once coincides with the period of ovulation.

To conclude, let me repeat that clinical experience has shown that coitus interruptus, practised over a long period, inevitably has undesirable repercussions on the mental and physical health of both man and wife. It is therefore not to be recommended.

Chapter 8
Vaginal Douching

Vaginal douching or 'injection" means flushing water or a chemical solution into the vagina in order to reach the posterior and anterior fornix (see diagram, p. 19).

Many women douche frequently, others occasionally, some rarely, and a few not at all. It's a matter of upbringing. Many consider a vaginal douche to be part of good feminine hygiene, particularly after intercourse or menstruation. However, according to modern gynecology, regular douching is not necessary.

The vaginal mucous membrane secretes a serous fluid which is slightly acid. It acts as a cleansing agent, sloughing off bacteria, dead cells, menstrual residue, etc. It contains millions of tiny organisms called the Döderlein bacilli, which destroy disease-producing germs and prevent their growth.

Physiologically speaking, the secretions produced by the vaginal lining are essential to good health, in much the same way as the gastric juices produced by the stomach. Vaginal douching eliminates the natural secretions.

.

Douching is not necessary after intercourse. The vagina is drained by the force of gravity and any seminal fluid which is not absorbed is therefore eliminated. The same is true of douching after using a diaphragm. If anything, it is the diaphragm that should be cleansed — but only after removal.

As for douching after menstruation, the whole idea is positively medieval. Some women look upon the menstrual flow as "bad blood" which the body must get rid of, rather than being simply the breakdown of the endometrium (mucous lining of the uterus) when nidation has not occurred. This is why they are inclined to douche when, in fact, it is not necessary.

Douching after intercourse with water and spermicidal products is not a sure means of contraception. Uninformed women do use it as such, but it should be realized that the only effective techniques for preventing fertilization and pregnancy are those used *before* intercourse : the condom, diaphragm, spermicidal creams and jellies.

Vaginal douching after intercourse for the purpose of entirely cleansing the vagina of seminal fluid ejaculated by the man during orgasm is totally ineffective, even if done several minutes later. The sperm cells have been launched from deep within the vagina, very close to the cervix. Considering the speed (one inch every eight minutes) at which sperm cells travel, they obviously pass through the cervix into the uterus almost immediately.

By the time douching with a spermicide takes place, the sperm cells have already entered the cervix. What is more the pressure from the douche actually

Vaginal Douche

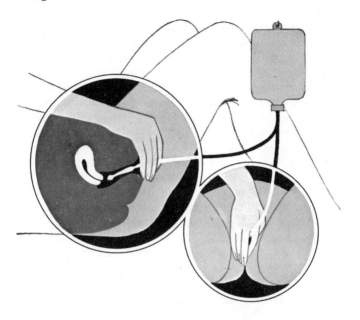

1 Fill the container with the prepared solution;
2 suspend the container about two feet above the body;
3 lie flat on the back in the bath, placing a folded towel beneath the small of the back in order to raise the hips slightly;
4 insert the nozzle into the vagina and let it fill slowly with the prepared solution;
5 hold the liquid in the vagina for several seconds (using the fingers to block the vaginal entrance) and then let it flow out;
6 repeat four or five times.

pushes some of the sperm cells into the uterus. Therefore there is a high risk of fertilization.

Consequently, vaginal douching is definitely not a means of contraception. It can be useful, however, if a diaphragm is mistakenly removed too soon or a condom torn or removed during intercourse. A spermicidal douche is better than nothing, but it would be safer to avoid the necessity for it altogether.

In the case of attempted coitus interruptus which is only partly successful, vaginal douching might help — again it is better than nothing. The seminal fluid may be deposited near the vaginal entrance or just inside, instead of higher up near the cervix, and a spermicidal douche might possibly prevent the sperm cells from continuing their journey.

I should emphasize, however, that vaginal douching with strong solutions in the hope of procuring an abortion is highly dangerous and sometimes fatal. All such preparations are harmful to the woman, and can destroy the mucous membrane or surrounding tissue, causing serious haemorrhage and possibly death.

Vaginal douching during pregnancy is permissible, as long as it is properly done. Then it will harm neither the mother nor the foetus, nor will it cause miscarriage. There is the risk, however, of washing away the beneficial prenatal secretions which prevent vaginal infections. Douching can also inhibit the g'ands which secrete a lubricating fluid during birth, thus easing the baby's passage through the birth canal.

It must be remembered that the cervix softens and dilates somewhat during pregnancy, and that a dou ching solution could pass through it into the uterus. It should only be done on a doctor's advice.

Strong antiseptics such as bichloride of mercury or Lysol irritate the vaginal walls and leave them open to infection. If no infection is present, a warm water douche is sufficient. The ideal temperature for the solution is as close to body temperature as possible, as overly hot water can burn the delicate genital tissue. Cold water can cause inflammation of the genital tract, or stop menstruation. The equipment used should be washed before and after.

As we have seen, vaginal douching is not a means of contraception, even if strong solutions are used. Its only effect is to damage or even destroy the mucous membrane of the vagina.

However, douching may be called for in specific treatments : e.g. for senile vaginitis (irritation or inflammation of the vagina in elderly women), which is treated by the internal application of a hormone cream. Douching is used the day after such treatment to wash away the cream. Routine douching is not necessary unless there is some medical reason for it.

Chapter 9
The Condom

The condom is a thin rubber sheath which covers the penis. There are various types of condoms which fall into two main categories : pre-lubricated and non-lubricated. The first is less irritating to the vaginal mucous membrane and less likely to cause secondary reactions after intercourse, such as vaginal itching and pain, or whitish discharge due to irritation by the condom.

Method

This contraceptive method is used by the man. The condom is unrolled onto the erect penis (see p. 85) just before vaginal penetration. It should not be done later, or just before ejaculation (expulsion of seminal fluid during male orgasm), because there may be sperm cells already present in the pre-coital fluid, and pregnancy may follow.

The condom catches and holds the ejaculated seminal fluid, thus preventing the sperm cells from entering the vagina, the uterus, and the Fallopian tubes. In other words, the risk of pregnancy is avoided. Most men have used a condom at some time. It makes possible a complete sexual act, enabling husband and wife to find fulfilment, even though they are deprived of direct genital contact. Some men find the condom uncomfortable, but it is still an ideal form of contraceptive in an emergency.

To be effective, of course, it must be used, and used properly, as described further on. If not, fertilization will occur. The male reproductive or sperm cells enter the vagina and swim up through the uterus to the Fallopian tubes. There, one successful sperm cell meets an egg and fertilizes it.

If the condom is covering the penis, it will catch the seminal fluid upon ejaculation. Therefore no sperm cell can reach the egg to fertilize it.

Description

The condom is made of a strong, thin rubber called latex. It is shaped like the finger of a glove, and adapts easily to the form of the erect penis. The open end is held by a rubber ring. The tip of the condom is sometimes shaped like a teat, to allow space for the seminal fluid once ejaculated. There are lubricated condoms, and these facilitate penetration.

The widespread use of the condom as a mechanical means of birth control goes back for centuries, and has continued even in this day and age of the hormone contraceptive pill.

The prophylactic sheath, as it is sometimes called, dates from ancient times. Archaeology has brought to light drawings and paintings on cave walls showing the use of the condom. The ancient Romans used animal bladders for this purpose. Even today there exist high-quality condoms made from sheep-gut. The Chinese made them of oiled tissue paper, and the Japanese developed a similar form.

The Condom

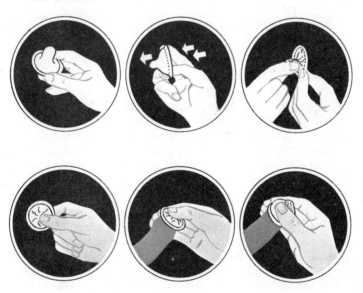

1 Air should be removed from the tip;
2 turn the tip inside out;
3 twist the tip into a spiral;
4 hold it so that the tip does not untwist;
5 place the condom on the penis;
6 gently unroll it.

The condom has long been used as a method of preventing venereal disease, particularly gonorrhoea. It is perhaps because of its association with these diseases or with socially illicit sex that the condom was considered unacceptable by many couples. The moralistic aspect has certainly influenced such couples greatly.

Proper Use of the Condom

The condom must be worn throughout the sexual act. Wives have consulted me for pregnancy, mystified because their husbands used a condom. The explanation in some cases is that the husband waited until just before ejaculation to use it. What he and his wife failed to realize was that, preparatory to sexual union, the Cowper's glands secrete a fluid which lubricates the male genital tract. This fluid may contain a few sperm cells which enter the vagina and swim up through the uterus to fertilize the waiting egg.

Questioning of the patient also reveals, in some cases, that after orgasm the husband delayed withdrawal longer than usual. Possibly the penis became less erect and the rubber ring at the opening fitted less tightly. In any case, attention should be paid to the rubber ring when withdrawing, to be sure that it does not slip, allowing some seminal fluid to escape.

If a good quality latex condom is used, it is unlikely to burst or tear unless roughly handled. A small amount of contraceptive cream may be used both inside and out, thus providing lubrication plus additional protection.

In spite of all precautions, accidents can happen. What can be done ? The woman can use a contraceptive cream applied with a vaginal applicator immediately after intercourse. If none is handy, a warm water douche, used immediately, may destroy many of the sperm cells. Whatever the method, speed is of the essence, as the sperm cells travel quickly. My advice would be always to have a contraceptive cream within reach.

Disadvantages

Married couples sometimes complain that the condom lessens physical satisfaction. I believe this is not so much the case now as it used to be. Clinical experiments have shown that physical sensation in the man is increased by placing a very small amount of contraceptive cream inside the condom. For the woman, a similar application inside the vagina has the same result. The cream also acts as a lubricant.

Sometimes a doctor will diagnose allergies caused by rubber or lubricating creams, but such reactions are not generally severe. If this is the case, however, it is advisable to use some other means of contraception, such as a diaphragm, IUD, hormone pill, etc.

In conclusion, the condom is a good mechanical contraceptive. This method is particularly useful for a couple after pregnancy, as long as they have no physical or mental reservations about using it.

Chapter 10
Chemical Spermicides

Spermicides come in the form of contraceptive jelly, cream or foam. They are acidic products, and all have the same purpose : to prevent the sperm cells from entering the uterus and fertilizing an egg in one of the Fallopian tubes. They are inserted high up in the vagina, near the cervix, where they block the progress of sperm cells and destroy them.

These jellies, creams and foams are not harmful to either man or woman. The foam is packaged in an aerosol can, but is introduced into the vagina with a special applicator, which is also used for the cream or jelly. The spermicide must be used before each separate act of intercourse.

One full applicator contains enough spermicide to ensure contraception. It is not necessary to douche after intercourse. As far as their effectiveness is concerned, vaginal spermicides offer better protection than such contraceptive measures as douching, suppositories, coitus interruptus or the rhythm method.

In principle, it is not necessary to use a diaphragm with these products, as their spermicidal action is effective on direct contact with the sperm cells. However, if a few sperm cells should succeed in penetrating the spermicidal barrier, particularly at the time of ovulation, there is a danger of pregnancy.

If a couple has definitely decided not to have any more children, the wife should ask her physician to prescribe a diaphragm, thus preventing any possible accident. The diaphragm (see Ch. 12 for full discussion) must be properly fitted by a doctor if it is to be effective, as the width between the end of the vagina (posterior fornix) and the pubic bone varies with each woman. To buy a diaphragm without knowing the correct size is to risk inadequate protection.

This mechanical contraceptive acts as a barrier, preventing the sperm cell's entry into the uterus. To be absolutely effective, it must be properly inserted, with spermicidal cream or jelly carefully applied to the inside, outside and around the rubber ring. If this is correctly done, a hermetically sealed barrier is created.

Various pharmaceutical companies have developed chemical spermicidal formulae which are odourless, colourless or whitish, do not stain sheets, do not interfere with the pleasure of intercourse, do not irritate the vaginal lining or cause inflammation of the cervix.

Vaginal Cream

This is a chemical substance containing a spermicide which immobilizes and destroys the sperm cells, thus acting as a contraceptive. There is, however, a ten to fifteen per cent risk of pregnancy. This

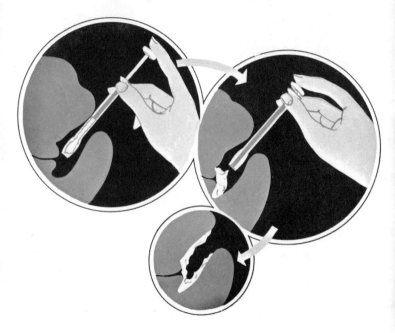

1 Insertion of cream, jelly or foam with special applicator.
2 The applicator is removed after being emptied.
3 The spermicide is spread around the vagina walls in the movements of intercourse.

form of contraception is short-term, and must be used immediately before intercourse. Some women make the mistake of douching right after intercourse rather than waiting at least eight hours.

Vaginal Foam

Vaginal foam is easily applied and is not harmful. It does not interfere with normal vaginal secretions, including the lubricating fluids, and does not irritate the vagina or penis.

It seems to be the simplest method of mechanical contraception, as it has very few side-effects. It is fairly effective, but is not as reliable as certain other methods. I would recommend it as a highly practical method for spacing births and delaying conception. For the couple which needs a totally effective contraceptive, the IUD or hormone pill are better choices.

Vaginal Jelly

Vaginal jelly is a chemical substance which acts as a barrier against sperm cells. It contains one or two ingredients which destroy sperm cells on contact. It has no effect on the cervix or the vagina. The jelly is inserted with a special applicator, just before each act of intercourse, and completely covers the cervix.

Chemical spermicides can cause eczema or irritation due to an allergic reaction. Such reactions are not usually severe, however.

In my view, these spermicides should be thought of as additional protection in conjunction with the use of a diaphragm, condom, or coitus interruptus.

Chapter 11
Antiseptic Vaginal Suppositories

Many women use vaginal suppositories as a contraceptive with, it would appear, a fair amount of success, although no precise statistics are available. These products have a spermicidal action, but I feel that luck must account partly for their effectiveness, such as it is. There is no doubt that they are not contraceptives in the real sense, such as spermicidal creams and foams, for example.

Use of Suppositories

The suppository should be removed from its protective plastic envelope with great care. It should be inserted high up in the vagina about ten minutes before intercourse, preferably in a lying down position. In the ten-minute interval body-heat dissolves the suppository completely, and an antiseptic coating is formed over the vaginal wall. The spermicidal ingredient immobilizes the sperm cells, in theory, but in my opinion it is not dependable. I would prefer to prescribe the hormone pill, IUD, or spermicidal foam.

As a means of birth control, suppositories are less reliable than creams or foams. In addition, medical science offers us completely reliable contraceptives, with the hormone pill heading the list. Next comes the IUD used with spermicidal foam ; the diaphragm with spermicidal cream ; and the condom with spermicidal foam. All are better than suppositories.

Some women feel that suppositories are easier to use and less bother than a diaphragm ; but their claim that they give equal protection is definitely false. For spacing births, suppositories *may* be useful, but for those who have finished having their family, they are inadequate.

These products, as I mentioned, have a certain spermicidal action, but not enough to be classed as effective contraceptives. It should be remembered that a spermicidal substance is one which can destroy sperm cells.

Deodorant Vaginal Suppositories

Many women use these small suppositories for their deodorant and antiseptic qualities. They say it makes them feel refreshed, more confident. I cannot help thinking that they are being overly zealous about genital hygiene.

The danger in using such products regularly is that the natural antiseptic products of the vagina may be interfered with, allowing harmful bacteria to grow unchecked, leading to fungoid growths and other undesirable conditions. I admit that women may feel "refreshed" when using them after menstruation, but again, as I pointed out in the section on douching, nature and the bath take care of normal vaginal cleanliness quite adequately.

The Vaginal Antiseptic Suppository in Place.

(Suppositories have a low contraceptive rating.)

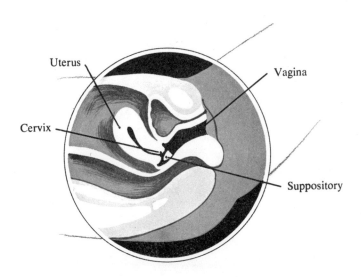

I have discussed suppositories mainly because many women believe that, in addition to being a deodorant, they are an effective form of contraception. Nothing could be more mistaken, and anyone who depends on these products is likely to have an unwanted pregnancy.

Chapter 12
The Diaphragm

The purpose of the diaphragm is to seal off the cervix — that is, the entrance to the uterus. A diaphragm is a saucer-shaped disc of soft, pliable rubber, attached to a flexible ring which holds it in shape.

Properly inserted in the vagina, it forms a hood over the cervix. The size required varies with each individual, and a gynecological examination by a physician is necessary to determine the precise measurements needed. The doctor also instructs his patient on the correct method of insertion and of checking its position.

The rubber hood does not seal off the uterus hermetically. Among the millions of sperm cells present in a single ejaculation, a few may therefore get around the diaphragm and work their way up through the uterus. To prevent this, the diaphragm is coated with a spermicidal jelly before insertion. It is also absolutely necessary to leave the diaphragm in place at least eight hours after intercourse.

This method has a considerable failure rate because of improper use : the diaphragm is either too small or too big, not correctly inserted, not used with a spermicidal cream, etc.

A diaphragm is preferable to the male condom, as it allows direct genital contact and complete sexual fulfilment. There are cases where either the man or woman feels inhibited by the presence of a diaphragm. Generally speaking, however, it is a good method of contraception if the directions are properly followed.

The diaphragm is not suitable for women suffering from genital infections. Those who are in good health from the gynecological standpoint may use it without

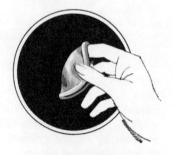

The diaphragm is compressed between the thumb and second finger to facilitate insertion.

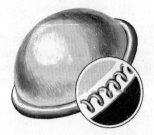

This diaphragm has a spring-coil ring which adapts well to the irregular contours of the vagina.

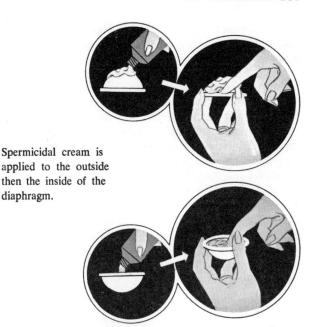

Spermicidal cream is applied to the outside then the inside of the diaphragm.

any harmful effects. As with the hormone pill, however, an annual medical checkup is advisable.

Nowadays diaphragms are manufactured with high-quality rubber which is very thin and pliable, and will not irritate the vaginal and uterine tissue.

As I mentioned earlier, the diaphragm is a good method of contraception. However, good methods sometimes do not work because the user has not mastered the technique. Women who are particularly tense may find it difficult or even impossible to use a diaphragm, as they are never confident and fear a possible pregnancy. Such women would be well-advised to ask their physician about the hormone pill, both for their own peace of mind and in the interests of a more rewarding sexual relationship.

Some women insert a diaphragm nightly in order to be protected if they have intercourse. This may affect a woman's sexual spontaneity.

In fact, all the traditional methods of birth control — the rhythm or Ogino method, condom, diaphragm, spermicidal jelly, etc. — have the same drawback: they interrupt the sex act in some way.

By contrast, the oral contraceptive or hormone pill has the advantage of not only giving total protection, but of preserving the spontaneity of the act of love. It is not a perfect solution, but it is the best now available.

However, if you prefer to use a diaphragm a visit to your doctor will be necessary. An internal pelvic examination will determine the exact size of diaphragm required.

Examination for Diaphragm

The physician inserts the index and second fingers in the vagina until they touch the posterior fornix or furthest end af the vagina. When the hand is lifted, it will touch the edge of the pubic bone. The thumb is used to mark the lower edge of the pubic bone in relation to the position of the two fingers, and this gives the measurement for the diaphragm.

This approximate measurement enables the physician to choose the diaphragm which matches the individual patient's dimensions, and which he then verifies by putting an actual diaphragm in place.

How to take
accurate measurements
for prescribing
a diaphragm.

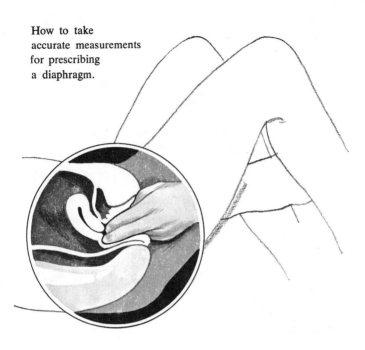

The measurement
is compared with
a specimen diaphragm.

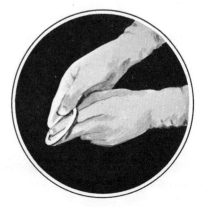

As an extra check, the physician tries larger and smaller ones as well. The correct diaphragm fits easily and causes no pressure.

How to Insert the Diaphragm

To begin with, a spermicidal cream is applied to the inside hollow and around the edge of the diaphragm, and then on the outside surface, in order to avoid irritating the vaginal lining. The cream seals the outer opening of the cervix.

Before inserting the diaphragm, the bladder must be emptied, either before going to bed or before intercourse. If intercourse is repeated, a full applicator of spermicidal cream should be inserted for extra protection (do *not* remove the diaphragm).

Can the diaphragm slip out of position? Not if it is properly inserted behind the pubic bone. It cannot be dislodged by body movements, changes in genital position, abdomino-vaginal contractions, urinating or bowel movements.

Certain women find the diaphragm uncomfortable. They should consult their doctor to check whether this discomfort is caused by a badly adjusted diaphragm, or one of incorrect size. Possibly there may be some malformation of the pelvis, or some internal vaginal abnormality such as cystocele (prolapse of the bladder into the vagina), anteflexion (tilting forward of the uterus), retroversion (tilting backward of the uterus), prolapse of the uterus, vaginal or uterine infection, or chronic constipation. Only a doctor is qualified to diagnose the problem.

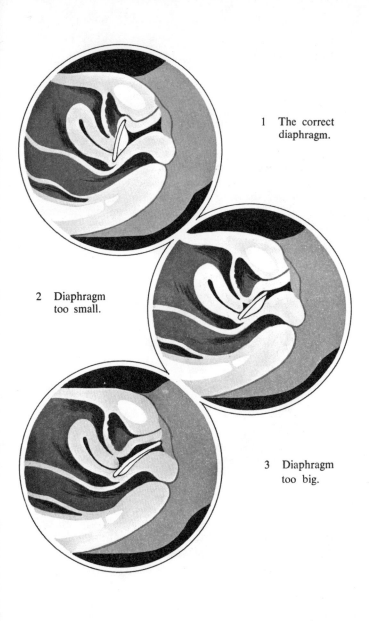

1 The correct diaphragm.

2 Diaphragm too small.

3 Diaphragm too big.

Removal

The diaphragm *must* be left in place for at least eight hours after intercourse. Some women like to douche (with boiled, lukewarm water) after removing it. Some gynecologists recommend using half the douche before removal, and half after.

The best method for removal is to hook the index finger under the ring of the diaphragm and draw it out gently. If it sticks, the user slips a finger between the vaginal wall and the edge of the diaphragm. This will make removal easier.

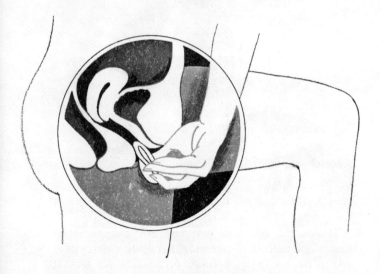

The correct diaphragm is inserted by the user. The diaphragm is compressed between the thumb and the middle finger.

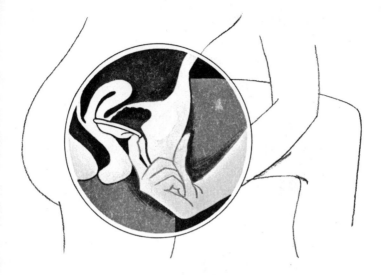

Once the diaphragm is inserted, the user pushes it
and then hooks it behind the pubic bone.

Keeping the Diaphragm Clean

Wash the diaphragm with warm water and a gentle
soap. Rinse and pat it dry. Do not boil it; do not
use an antiseptic solution.

If you are not sure that you are inserting your
diaphragm correctly, you should consult your doctor.
Otherwise you may become pregnant. An annual
visit to your doctor is recommended in any case, as
with women who use the hormone pill. The required
size of diaphragm may change for various reasons:

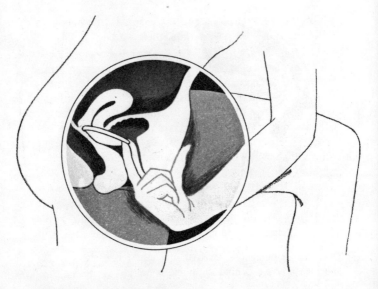

Removal of the diaphragm eight hours or more after intercourse. The index finger is hooked under the nearest edge of the diaphragm ring.

for example, after giving birth there is usually a variation of several millimeters in pelvic measurements, and therefore a new diaphragm is necessary.

The diaphragm is a relatively popular form of contraception, and there is no denying its effectiveness when used correctly. However, many women entering their forties have switched from the diaphragm to the hormone pill. Although the diaphragm gave adequate protection, they prefer to use a contraceptive which offers complete security, since pregnancy is particularly to be avoided at their age.

Doctors are frequently consulted by women who use the diaphragm but have become pregnant, thus losing confidence in this method. Clinical examination shows that it is almost always the fault of the user, not the contraceptive. Sometimes she doesn't use it during her sterile days; perhaps it is not properly inserted, or not left in long enough after intercourse. Possibly she has not visited her doctor regularly in order to check possible change in size, particularly after a pregnancy.

These days, women have a variety of contraceptives available. Some become confused and don't know which to choose. It is my opinion that the choice of contraceptive prescribed depends on a woman's stage of life with respect to the genital organs. Around forty, for example, the hormone pill is the most suitable method of contraception, because it is one hundred per cent effective. At this age, too, women often require some hormone replacement therapy.

The pill is also prescribed for couples wishing to space out births. It is prescribed, after gynecological examination, for the young woman whose education is not finished, and for whom an unwanted pregnancy could ruin both career and future. There is no doubt that, for the present, the hormone pill is better than all other contraceptives.

Nevertheless, a fair number of women adapt well to using the diaphragm, and do not find it bothersome or frustrating. So much the better : they will continue to use this method, since it suits them and poses no problems.

Chapter 13
The Intra-Uterine Device

The intra-uterine device is a mechanical contraceptive which is inserted in the uterus by a special instrument. A physician must perform the insertion. The IUD prevents pregnancy. Once inserted, it can remain in place until the woman wishes to conceive.

The IUD is usually made of flexible white plastic which sets up no adverse reaction in body tissues. The shapes which seem to be most effective, since they cause fewer problems and side-effects, are the coil and the loop. The question remains : is the IUD as effective as the hormone pill ?

When speaking of effectiveness, one must take every aspect into consideration, including the patient's responsibility. The pill is considered one hundred per cent effective, on condition that the user does not forget to take it — not even for one day. The IUD has a two to four per cent risk of failure. However, once it is inserted, there can be no question of mistakes or omissions. In the field of contraception, the pill and the IUD offer the greatest security.

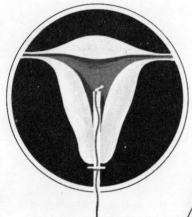

Metal probe in uterus. (Insertion is performed by a gynecologist.) The IUD is inside the probe.

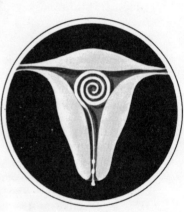

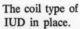

The coil type of IUD in place.

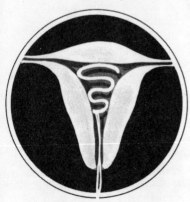

The loop type of IUD in place.

It should be noted that there is a period of adaptation by the uterus to the IUD, which is, after all, a foreign body. Initially the menstrual cycle may be slightly changed. Some women have a heavier flow for a day or two during the first and second periods. It is normal for flecks of blood to appear after the gynecologist has inserted the IUD and also a few days before the next menstruation.

Are there cases where the IUD should not be used? Most definitely. What are they? Acute or subacute diseases of the uterus or its appendages (ovaries, Fallopian tubes); fibroid tumours of the uterus (benign growths on the uterine muscle), particularly those beneath the mucous lining; menorrhagia (excessive blood-flow during menstruation); any vaginal bleeding of abnormal or undiagnosed origin; inflammation of the cervix (severe or chronic); and suspicion of cancer of the uterus or cervix.

How does the IUD work? We haven't really any scientifically proven explanation. It is thought that its presence increases muscular activity to the point of preventing or interfering with the meeting of sperm and egg; or perhaps of preventing nidation (i.e. the implantation of the fertilized egg in the mucous lining of the uterus). A more recent theory suggests that the presence of a foreign body in the uterus releases a defensive substance (a sort of antibody) which may paralyze the sperm cells.

Since the IUD is a foreign body in the uterus, the muscle is more easily activated or irritated, and the IUD can, in some cases, be rejected by means of strong uterine contractions.

Some women are afraid that the IUD might harm a baby, should they conceive in spite of its presence — although this rarely happens. The foetus will not be harmed, because the baby develops within its own protective sac of amniotic fluid. The IUD usually comes out after the birth.

A few women are continually worried that the IUD may slip out. This can easily be checked by inserting the middle finger in the vagina until it touches the "beads" or plastic string attached to the IUD.

Why don't doctors prescribe the IUD for women who have not borne children? There is no medical reason, strictly speaking. It is easier, however, and causes less discomfort, to insert an IUD in a uterus which has already been enlarged by pregnancy. In addition, it would seem that the larger uterus rarely rejects the IUD, whereas the virgin uterus may do so more readily.

I should repeat here that the IUD is not one hundred per cent effective — no mechanical device is. There is always a slight risk of pregnancy, and a woman should realize this before making any decision.

Can the IUD be inserted at any time during the menstrual cycle? No. It is preferable to do it during menstruation, thereby reducing the risk of insertion when pregnancy has already begun.

Women who have just had a baby wonder how soon the IUD can be inserted. Not immediately, as the uterus would reject it at once. Several weeks must elapse before consulting a physician to have the IUD inserted.

I have had patients who have used the IUD for several years consult me because they suddenly fear it can cause cancer of the uterus. There is no foundation for such fear. The IUD does not cause cancer. Although some authorities believe that continual irritation of an organ is a possible element in causing cancer, these same authorities are all agreed that this does not apply to the interior of the uterus. Since the uterus lining rids itself of its cells each month, there is no danger of prolonged irritation by the IUD, and therefore no reason to fear cancer of the uterus as a result.

You may have heard about a new method, by which a small device is inserted into the uterus, where hormones are released. It is still in the experimental stage, and is similar to the methods where hormones are absorbed by mouth or by injection. The hormones pass from the uterus through the vagina walls and into the blood stream. This method is not developed for prescription as yet.

How is the coil IUD inserted? To begin with, the physician examines the physical condition of the reproductive organs, particularly the form and position of the uterus, and checks for pregnancy.

The physician then inserts a speculum (a surgical instrument for dilating orifices of the body), and introduces the probe into the cervix with great care, in order to avoid any injury to the interior of the uterus. The insertion is done very gently, without

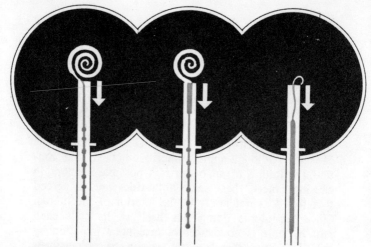

The IUD is unrolled into the intra-uterine probe by the gynecologist.

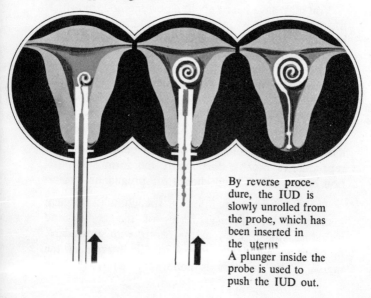

By reverse procedure, the IUD is slowly unrolled from the probe, which has been inserted in the uterus
A plunger inside the probe is used to push the IUD out.

undue pressure, and under the most sterile conditions possible.

Wearing sterile gloves, the physician inserts the IUD or coil into the uterine probe and directs it towards the cervix and the fundus of the uterus. The IUD is pushed out by the metal plunger in the probe, resuming its coil shape within the uterus. The probe and plunger are withdrawn, and the physician cuts the end of the IUD, leaving a plastic string or two beads hanging outside the cervix, in order to facilitate removal of the IUD when desired.

The IUD can be inserted by a doctor around the fifth week after birth. It can remain in place indefinitely, or be carefully removed by a physician should any severe side-effects occur or should a further pregnancy be decided upon.

The doctor instructs his patient how to make a weekly check on whether or not the IUD is in place. If she feels the beads near the cervix, all is well; but if the smooth portion of the IUD is felt, it has slipped out of position. The woman should wash her hands thoroughly before each check.

Cramps may be felt after the IUD has been inserted. Slight bleeding may occur during the first few days, and the first two periods may be earlier, longer, and with a heavier flow than usual. An annual examination is necessary.

Chapter 14
The Hormone Pill

The hormone pill is an effective, medically approved method of contraception. It prevents ovulation and stops the uterus from preparing for nidation — that is, from providing shelter and nourishment for a fertilized egg. The pill is taken each evening during a twenty-one day period, beginning with the fifth day of the cycle for the first treatment. After this, the user stops for seven days and then resumes treatment. This method is used by a great many married women, mothers, and women who are nearing menopause.

This is the best method of contraception known, providing virtually absolute protection. The husband and wife are freed from the nuisance of preparation before intercourse. No foreign body is present, and the couple are not subject to the psychological or physical difficulties which may arise in using other methods. In fact, the hormone pill seems to help overcome psycho-sexual inhibitions. Only one thing is needed : a good memory. The user must take the pill every day.

A couple who have had a happy marital and sexual relationship for ten or fifteen years cannot cut off their erotic impulses merely because they have finished having children. Like other contraceptives, the hormone pill enables such couples to continue their fulfilling sex life.

The psychosomatic and mental side-effects of abstinence are thus avoided — whether such abstinence is through fear of unwanted pregnancy or feelings of guilt connected with the use of a mechanical contraceptive. The ailments caused by abstinence can vary from indigestion, heart and respiratory ailments, troubles in the muscles, joints or pelvis, to depression and even psychosis.

The pill is a modern miracle which helps couples to live a healthy, serene, and emotionally secure life. Their physical union remains happy, well-balanced and durable.

The pill can be described as absolute protection — or very nearly ; but you must follow the directions to the letter, and consult your physician if there is any sign of an adverse reaction. A yearly visit to your gynecologist must be made without fail.

Why Family Planning ?

Let us look at the basic question : why should we limit the number of births ? In order to prevent the population of our country from increasing too rapidly ? Overpopulation is a critical issue in many countries and it is rapidly becoming so in North America. To lower the number of abortions ? This is a humane and valid reason, since abortion is a

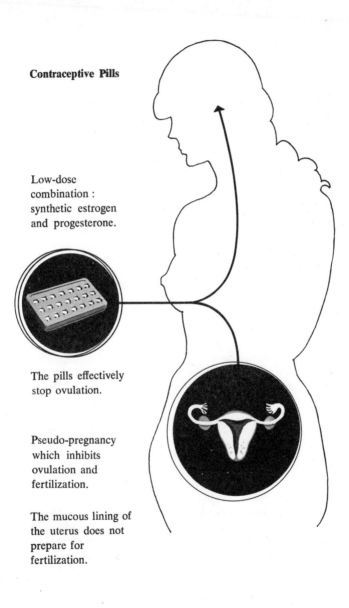

Contraceptive Pills

Low-dose
combination :
synthetic estrogen
and progesterone.

The pills effectively
stop ovulation.

Pseudo-pregnancy
which inhibits
ovulation and
fertilization.

The mucous lining of
the uterus does not
prepare for
fertilization.

Natural Hormones During Pregnancy:

Progesterone and estrogen.

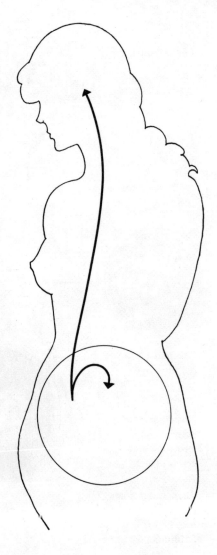

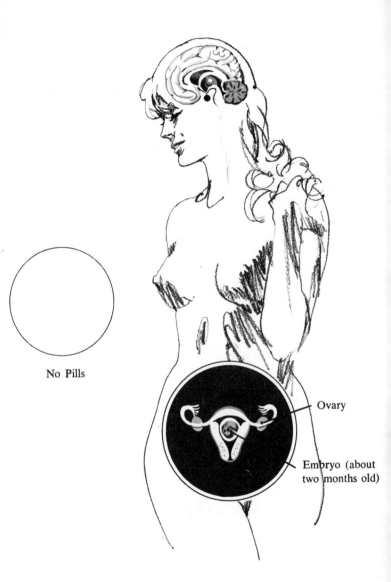

No Pills

Ovary

Embryo (about
two months old)

drastic measure which is resorted to all too often. In the majority of cases, abortion is detrimental to the mental and physical health of the woman concerned.

In the last few years the medical profession has tended to favour contraceptives which prevent ovulation, especially the hormone pill, with a view to eliminating the resort to abortion. Such an outlook is desirable, since it solves many problems — often very serious ones.

For example, the problem of unwanted pregnancies is acute. Resorting to the use of litmus paper or basal temperature to determine the fertile period is practically useless as a means of contraception, as these methods only apply to a woman with perfect hormone balance. For the majority of women whose periods are not always regular, the doctor prescribes the hormone pill which inhibits ovulation and makes family planning genuinely possible. The couple will also have a more satisfactory sex life through using the pill, in comparison with such methods as vaginal douching, vaginal cream or foam, the diaphragm, condom or coitus interruptus.

Women of Roman Catholic faith are often upset at the thought of using the pill, feeling that to do so conflicts with the dictates of conscience. Will the Church one day free them from this moral dilemma ? I most sincerely hope so, both for their own physical and mental well-being, and in the interests of a happy home.

A family cannot live in harmony unless the couple and their children are well-balanced mentally and physically. This cannot be achieved if responsibilities are overwhelming. Family planning is a means of preventing marital and family breakdown.

A doctor respects a couple's freedom of choice, and will not refuse to prescribe the pill if the mental and physical condition of the wife is normal. Every woman has the right to marry, make a home, and have one, two or three children, depending on her own wishes and in agreement with her husband. Together, the couple consider their resources : health, responsibilities, economic situation, and the broader social and ecological circumstances. Then they themselves make the decision. To impose abstinence for purposes of family planning would be inhumane. Sooner or later sexual deprivation affects the mental and physical health of a couple.

Couples who use the contraceptive pill for the first year or two of marriage have a better opportunity to adapt to one another emotionally, sexually and in terms of their personalities. The pill is also prescribed when hormone balance is faulty. Couples adopt this method, too, under medical supervision, after their planned family has arrived.

Case Histories

A young woman suffered from nervous tension during her pregnancy. The baby — a girl — arrived in good health. A month after, when she consulted me for her check-up, I asked her if she wished to discuss contraceptive methods. "No," she replied, "that won't be necessary." I was naturally curious and asked why. "My husband wants a divorce," was the answer.

During her pregnancy this young woman had shown no interest in sex, as she did not think it important. Her husband accused her of never having truly loved him. I took the opportunity of pointing out how self-centred her attitude had been, as well as making her realize her lack of understanding and complete ignorance of the real meaning of marriage.

She consulted me again three years later. By this time she had remarried, and was very happy. She thanked me for having opened her eyes to the psychology of married life, which she had been very careful to respect from the start of her second marriage.

Women often lose the desire for sexual intercourse during pregnancy. One of the most frequent contributing factors to separation and divorce, in cases where the wife is pregnant at marriage or shortly after, is precisely the stress and constraint imposed by an early pregnancy.

These young couples have not had the time or opportunity to learn to live comfortably together before actively undertaking the responsibilities and strains of a family. Depending on how mature they are, one or two years of using a contraceptive would have enabled them to adapt better emotionally and sexually, as well as to adjust their personalities to the give-and-take of daily life together.

It is a fact that some men resent sharing their wife's attention with their own offspring. They may sulk when the young mother is nursing or otherwise caring for the baby. She in turn is at a loss what to do. Decidedly, parenthood has come too soon.

Young couples such as these have not had time to acquire the maturity which would have enabled them to understand what is implied by parenthood and its obligations. Here again, the use of a completely sure method, for at least two years, would have benefited their emotional well-being.

A woman is often subject to physical and emotional upsets from the beginning of pregnancy. Nausea, for example, may occur during the first ten or twelve weeks, to the point where even the smell of food is revolting and preparation of meals distasteful.

The woman whose early pregnancy is unwanted inevitably finds things difficult. She loses her enthusiasm, is no longer interested in various activities, and sometimes undergoes fairly severe depression throughout the prenatal period or even after the birth. The young, inexperienced husband, lacking the maturity to deal with such a situation in marriage, feels totally bewildered. It's unfortunate that he didn't seek advice about contraceptive methods.

Financial Problems

Financial problems are a stumbling block for many a young couple. Doctor's appointments, medication during pregnancy, hospital costs and fees for the delivery — they all add up. This financial drain often comes on top of steep monthly payments on furnishings for the new home, and perhaps on the car as well. Then the wife, who is usually working, is obliged to stop around the sixth or seventh month.

After the baby is born, the couple's way of life is somewhat altered, to say the least. They can't seem to see a movie when they want to, play bridge with friends when planned, or do anything enjoyable. The baby is sick or colicky, and they have to stay at home. They can't get away for weekends, either. Finally, they begin to feel frustrated, disappointed and confined. Invariably, fights occur, and marriage breakdown begins. What is needed to overcome all the strain and inconvenience of parenthood is an opportunity for emotional and sexual adaptation, plus a great deal of love and understanding.

The young mother often has conflicting feelings about her baby. When he cries, when her sleep is interrupted night after night, when she wakes each morning to a mountain of diapers, she becomes unsure about loving him.

Violent resentment towards the situation — which makes her irritable, unbalanced and generally upset — plus the doubts about her love for the child, cause subconscious guilt feelings. Finally, she becomes a nervous wreck, would like to dump the whole business of motherhood, and refuses to listen to reason. Her problem has got the better of her.

There is no doubt that family planning and contraception are beneficial to the well-being of both man and woman, and the couple as a unit.

The contraceptive hormone pill creates bodily conditions similar to those of pregnancy. Ovulation stops ; the breasts are heavier ; and there is a tendency to gain weight if food intake is not watched. Some women complain of a decrease in sexual desire.

A few women even claim that sexual desire disappears. I had a young woman consult me in tears on this point. She had used the hormone pill for two years. "I always enjoyed making love with my husband," she told me. "It was a very precious moment for both of us. Now I absolutely refuse. What's happening to me?"

In her case I advised stopping the pill and using some other contraceptive method: diaphragm, IUD, or condom. Two weeks later she had regained her former ardour. A wise woman does not allow herself to be overwhelmed by such a problem.

Contraception in Early Marriage

Is it unhealthy? No; on the contrary, it benefits the young couple. There are several factors to be considered, one being the wife's age. Preferably, pregnancy should occur after the age of twenty-one, because mentally and physically the woman is stronger. If the couple's financial situation is unsure, again it would be better to wait. If the husband is still at university and his wife is working to help put him through, then they should wait. In each of these cases an early pregnancy could cause real marital problems. The added strain of parenthood may push the couple apart, lead to frigidity, or end in divorce.

How long should parenthood be delayed? Not too long. If a young husband becomes too accustomed to being the centre of his wife's love and attention for too many years, he may find it difficult to share her with another — even his own child.

Common sense, co-operation, self-discipline and judgment are necessary for truly helpful family planning.

Erotic Pleasure

For many married couples, the hormone pill greatly enhances sexual relations. The possibility of completely spontaneous love-making, plus the lack of tension and fear of pregnancy, create a more relaxed and voluptuous atmosphere. The older methods of contraception tend to diminish this carefree approach to love-making, whereas with the pill many couples find they make love more often.

A New Problem

The hormone pill has created a problem for people with a low level of sexual desire — a fact of which they may have been unaware. The Ogino or rhythm method suited them, as the permitted time for intercourse was reduced to five or six days in each menstrual cycle. They are perhaps thirty, thirty-five or forty — the best years in one's sexual life — get on well together, have enough leisure and not too many problems with the children. They have no serious financial difficulties and, in short, life is very pleasant.

Then the subject of the pill comes up — perhaps the wife suffers from menstrual irregularity. In any case, they discuss the pill with their doctor. This is the perfect time to begin such treatment, the wife finding it very inconvenient to have perhaps two periods a month, or one very long period. Mechanical methods of contraception are unattractive for this couple, as they are not in the habit of using them and the thought is distasteful.

After taking the pill for several months, the wife becomes far more passionately attracted to her husband than even in early marriage. She appreciates her new-found liberty, whereas the husband, paradoxically, sometimes rejects it. How? He complains of tiredness, headache, watches the late-late show, raids the fridge or reads a book.

Instead of approaching the marriage-bed with enthusiasm, he drags his feet. The demand for love-making is too much for him. His wife tries to fire his emotions, to change his ideas about sex.

The Wife's Ingenuity

Such a situation may seem comic to the outsider, but for those involved it can be tragic. Suddenly their accepted sexual balance is disrupted, and if the wife is to make her husband's enthusiasm equal hers she must proceed with care.

It would be all too easy to make the husband feel inadequate in the face of the wife's new and greater demands. For her part, unless she is an understanding woman, she may feel angered and rejected. Badly handled, the situation may lead to resentment, jealousy, hate and a desire for vengeance.

Remember, more flies are caught with honey than vinegar. It is the wife's task to encourage her husband and lead him tenderly towards a more frequent enjoyment of intercourse.

The husband will respond to his wife's understanding and encouragement, although it may take time.

A Question of Habit

A number af married couples make love at a definite time, or times, during the week. By tacit agreement they organize their lives to provide an opportunity for being alone together and undisturbed. They look forward to it and are ready when the time comes. Suppose, however, that the wife is not entirely satisfied with using the diaphragm, although in spite of the inconvenience they achieve a fairly high degree of mutual fulfilment.

In the hope of having greater sexual enjoyment the couple consider the contraceptive pill. They perhaps have visions of long, languorous nights of love-making. The wife believes that her husband will leap joyfully into bed each night in order to make the most of her new-found freedom. To her immense surprise, such is not the case. The husband preferred things as they were.

He begins to feel that he is a poor specimen of a lover with a very deficient sense of romance. Even his eyesight seems to have deteriorated to the point where his wife's charms leave him cold. How could he have changed so?

The answer is that the era ushered in by the contraceptive pill has totally unsettled him. Accustomed to a predictable sexual routine, he can't adapt to the unexpected. Change is inimical to him, and forcing him to assume a more romantic attitude may give rise to genuine problems. This type of man finds comfort in knowing ahead of time what his love-making activities will be. He likes to know that he will have intercourse on a certain day. It gives him confidence, a sense of well-being and vigour. More men than one would think feel this way. The pill poses a real dilemma for them. My recommendation would be to avoid placing such a man under a strain which might prove too much for his self-esteem. If the wife truly wishes her husband's love-making to be more frequent and impromptu, she will need a remarkable talent for gentle persuasion and tact, and must be prepared to carry on the treatment for a long time.

To sum up, I would say that if the pill can benefit both partners in marriage, it is performing a great service.

Why Not a Pill for Men?

Why is it the woman who has to take the pill and not the man? Early research was directed towards suppressing female ovulation rather than stopping sperm development, because it was far easier to accomplish. The former procedure was already used frequently in treating dysmenorrhea (painful or difficult menstruation) and endometriosis (change in appearance of cells of the uterine lining, resulting in menstrual unbalance).

In addition, men are far more susceptible to psychological reactions affecting their sexual activity than women. Their sense of masculinity in relation to the sex act is easily threatened, whereas women's sense of femininity is not. Men easily become impotent, and even though they traditionally assume the aggressive role in sex, are extremely sensitive to the slightest insult to their manhood.

When a woman assumes a markedly aggressive attitude after years of playing the more usual role in love-making, a real problem is created. This new attitude is a direct result of her release from fear of pregnancy. She takes pleasure in sex, is ardently interested and often violently aggressive in her demands. Some husbands may find such behaviour fascinating, but others only become frustrated, afraid, distressed and even impotent.

Typical Case Histories

A lively, talkative salesman, interested in a variety of activities such as hunting, fishing, golf, tennis, etc., and proud of what he regarded as his sexual prowess, blamed his fairly frail wife for their infrequent love-making (once every six weeks). Finally, he asked her to use the pill so that intercourse might take place in a more relaxed atmosphere. She agreed, and once her fear of pregnancy was removed she began to enjoy sex for the first time in her life. However, they did not have intercourse more often than before, and it became evident that the infrequency of sexual relations was really due to the husband.

Another couple had a paradoxical sexual relationship which only became apparent to them when the wife began taking the contraceptive pill. Before, his wife's frigidity had been a target for the husband's aggression (pseudo-aggression). He complained of not getting enough sex. In fact, he didn't really want more. The wife, now no longer frigid, is unsatisfied. The husband continues to live with his fears, and the wife thinks of looking elsewhere for satisfaction.

Sometimes the husband's reaction takes the form of jealousy. In the case of a wife who decided to use the pill after her third pregnancy, a definite change in the husband's behaviour became evident after a few months. He was overbearing, moody, suspicious, hostile, and less interested in sex. He feared the possibility of his wife's seeking sexual satisfaction outside marriage, accused her of driving him mad, and began to threaten physical violence.

Contraception obliges some men to face up to their real sexual potential. All too often, since the advent of the pill, men and women have panicked on this subject, driving themselves into a state of depression.

The hormone pill seems to have given woman a genuine feeling of sexual equality, so that she not only actively participates during the act, but feels confident enough to initiate it. This amounts to overthrowing most of our subconscious ideas about sex, inherited from the Victorian era, and has resulted in a veritable orgasmic explosion among women. The feminine mystique has deserted the marriage-bed. Through the pill, women have become more interested and aggressive in sex. This poses a genuine problem for many men, who only looked for personal satisfaction from sex and can't adapt to the sexual change in their wives.

The pill eliminates unwanted pregnancies. Career women can easily put off motherhood. One totally bewildered husband told me, "She doesn't want any children — never talks about it. It makes me very sad. She seems totally self-centred, and I find her selfishness most unpleasant." This woman lived only for her career, thought only about money, freedom and her self-respect. Such a case is unusual, but very difficult for the husband.

The hormone pill is an excellent contraceptive and has the added benefit of possibly increasing the wife's interest in sex. But it contains no ingredient for relieving marital stress, no magic substance enabling a husband to perform beyond his individual sexual powers. If the husband is willing to accept the wife's increased sexual desire, and if she, in turn, respects his sensitivity, their love-life may indeed blossom. The pill forces husbands and wives to come to terms with their own sexuality, and it can lead to a more mature marriage.

Chapter 15
Male and Female Sterilization

Female Sterilization

I have had women between the ages of twenty-five and forty consult me about sterilization. They do not want any more children. Often they are using mechanical contraceptives with which they are dissatisfied, or which they do not trust. Several have been taking the contraceptive pill for some years, but fear long-range effects. They are therefore seeking a permanent solution to the problem of contraception.

Others ask the doctor to persuade their mate to undergo vasectomy, or male sterilization, claiming that they have done enough for him and that another operation would be detrimental to their health. They are often right in this respect. What does the husband say? All too often he refuses. So the woman resigns herself once more to surgery, in the hope that the operation will lead to a better-balanced, more harmonious marriage.

Is female sterilization legal? Is a healthy organ involved? If so, does it amount to mutilation? Not always. There are valid medical reasons for it.

One is always reluctant to operate on healthy Fallopian tubes. In addition, the woman who wants sterilization now may change her mind later, blaming the surgeon for having deprived her of the possibility of having children. If men and women weren't in the habit of making accusations, things would be much simpler. As it is, a committee of physicians is required to take such a decision, and each case is carefully studied.

Various Considerations

Women do divorce or become widows and subsequently remarry. The future husband may want children — who knows? Or the new wife, once more in love, may wish to have a child by her new husband. What then?

When disease is present, the surgeon performs a salpingectomy (removal of a Fallopian tube) without question, because he must. Unless there is a valid medical reason, he will not perform a female or male sterilization. Such reasons include : several children already ; one or two difficult Caesarian sections ; general fatigue ; cardio-vascular troubles ; chronic pulmonary ailments such as asthma, emphysema, etc. ; circulatory difficulties in the lower limbs ; severe reaction to the pill ; chronic anxiety and depression, etc.

According to some specialists, successful reversal of surgical sterilization is rare. Very, very rare, I would say.

By contrast, there is a twenty-five per cent chance of surgically re-establishing fertility in the case of male vasectomy, according to certain urologists. I

Surgical Female Sterilization

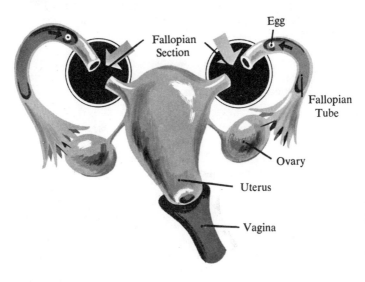

The Surgeon's Procedure

1 Laboratory (abdominal incision);
2 section (severing) of the Fallopian tubes;
3 ligation of the severed ends.

find this percentage rather high myself. It is better to consider sterilization as a permanent step, both for men and women, in order to avoid serious disappointment in the future.

If you are considering it, you should first discuss the problem thoroughly with your family doctor. You should not be afraid to tell him frankly your feelings, anxieties, fears, and marital difficulties. For some, psychotherapy is the answer for achieving freedom from inhibition, including fear of pregnancy (although I am speaking here of those women who have never had children). For others, the family doctor will study the case carefully, taking into account the medical reasons, and submit it to a medical board which will decide for or against surgical sterilization. You will have done all that is required of you and can proceed with a clear conscience.

Various women want permanent sterilization because of psychological problems. Are you suffering from a rejection of your femininity? Were you brought up by a mother who really did not want children? Do you regret having had children? Do you feel incapable of being a mother? Do you lack self-confidence? A psychiatric examination is called for.

The whole question is a delicate one, particularly because surgical sterilization in women is, to all intents and purposes, irreversible. The same is virtually true for men. So think about it seriously!

Male Sterilization (Vasectomy)

For some couples, vasectomy is a suitable form of contraception. But be careful of damaging psychological side-effects !

What is vasectomy ? It is the severing (or "section") of the vas deferens and ligation of the severed ends. Sperm cells are thus prevented from travelling from the testicles to the point of ejaculation near the urethra. Any blockage of these ducts, whether by surgery, traumatism or disease, causes sterility.

To obtain vasectomy there must be a valid medical reason : physical, emotional or mental. In addition, the wife must also be willing. It is preferable for the patient to have had one or two children, in order to prevent any post-operative psychological reactions. Most vasectomies are permanent, therefore sterility is a clinically established fact. However, vasectomy in no way affects a man's masculine traits or his capacity to make love.

Men who have undergone vasectomy and have subsequently divorced may regret having had the operation. The chances of a second marriage producing children are highly unlikely. Although the ducts may be repaired surgically, fertility does not often return. Vasectomy is a simple operation, but the reverse procedure is not so easy. As one urologist has said, "Vasectomy is the simplest operation in the field of urology." The complications arise from a sharp change in the patient's mental attitude, marked by a strong feeling of regret at having had the operation.

One occasionally hears of a wife becoming pregnant after her husband has had a vasectomy. What explains it? The severed ducts have become joined again, allowing the sperm cells to pass through from the testicles. Urologists call it a spontaneous re-channelling of the seminal ducts. Another extremely rare occurrence is the existence of an extra seminal duct which is not detected by the surgeon. Fertilization is therefore possible, although medical literature only gives a few instances of this phenomenon.

Both husbands and wives have admitted achieving a high degree of sexual fulfilment after vasectomy. Why? Because fear of pregnancy is totally overcome, and the need for mechanical contraceptives, which may affect spontaneity in intercourse, is eliminated. Some men have an unfortunate reaction, however, becoming emotionally upset — a sort of defence mechanism against an unconscious feeling of castration.

The man who unconsciously thinks of vasectomy as a form of castration over-reacts in order to bolster his masculinity, his virility. The wife and the marriage may suffer greatly as a result. Generally speaking, however, the negative aspects of vasectomy are usually compensated for by the emotional and sexual benefits to the couple and their marriage.

What exactly is the operation? Vasectomy is simple, lasts about twenty minutes, and is often performed with a local anaesthetic. The surgeon makes an incision of about half to one inch long in the scrotum; the spermatic cord is exposed, and a small portion of the vas deferens is isolated and severed. The ends are tied off (ligation), after which the skin is closed and sutured with catgut.

Some men want a vasectomy in order to limit their families and spare their wives a further pregnancy. Others choose it because their wives have

Surgical Male Sterilization

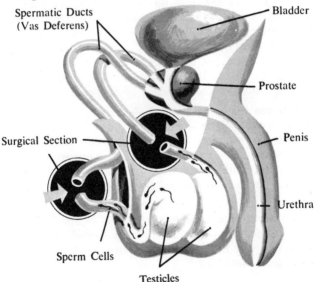

Spermatic Ducts (Vas Deferens)

Bladder

Prostate

Surgical Section

Penis

Urethra

Sperm Cells

Testicles

The Surgeon's Procedure

1 Incision in scrotum (about one inch) ;
2 section (severing) of vas deferens ;
3 ligation of the severed ends ;
4 incision in scrotum stitched with catgut.

been advised by a doctor that another pregnancy might be dangerous. Some men are willing to undergo vasectomy rather than permit their wives to have the analogous female operation, because in the woman it involves major surgery (laparotomy, meaning abdominal incision).

Once they have undergone vasectomy, men are generally less tense, and do not feel they have lost their masculinity. The fact that sexual intercourse is normally resumed several days after the operation eliminates fears about their virility. A contraceptive should be used for six weeks after the vasectomy, in order to check the seminal fluid microscopically at least twice for the presence of sperm cells.

It seems that intercourse is more frequent during the first year after vasectomy. Later it gradually resumes the pre-operative pattern. Some men claim that vasectomy gives them more control over ejaculation, and therefore greater sexual fulfilment. Whether or not this is purely imaginary, who can say?

The wives of men who have had a vasectomy are usually freed from restraint by the knowledge that pregnancy will not follow intercourse, and their sex life benefits accordingly.

Male sterilization is undertaken when both husband and wife are in full agreement, and in consideration of the reasons given for their decision. The case is also reviewed by a medical board, which usually includes a urologist, a psychiatrist, a specialist in internal medicine, and in some cases, a religious or moral adviser.

Chapter 16
Resistance to Contraception

Many women resort to highly unreliable methods for preventing pregnancy. Why, I cannot for the life of me understand, since they do not want any more children. Then again, many married — and unmarried — women are desperately afraid of intercourse without protection, but still won't take the necessary precautions. A greater paradox can scarcely be imagined! Some even have a mechanical or some other form of contraceptive available, but refuse to use it. I am not speaking here of cases where opposition is due to religious or ethical scruples.

Take the case of a young unmarried woman. She needs fully reliable protection. An unwanted pregnancy will make her future very difficult, to say nothing of upsetting her emotional relationship with the man involved, whom she may lose as a result.

Then there is the woman who has been warned by her doctor to avoid further pregnancy on health grounds. She obstinately refuses to use a sure method of contraception, gets "caught," and begins to ask around for the name of an abortionist. What nonsense ! Why adopt such an attitude ? Because for these women, the use of a mechanical contraceptive or the hormone pill creates greater anxiety than the fear of pregnancy.

Take the truly sad case af a young woman of twenty-three, divorced because an unhealthy dependence on her parents prevented her from whole-heartedly devoting herself to her husband as a normal wife would. Later she meets a patient, attentive man. He gives her to understand that he is not interested in prudish women, and in fear of losing him she consults a doctor who prescribes a diaphragm. Once home again, she bursts into tears, and subsequently undergoes severe mental depression. Psychiatric examination reveals that this woman has been subject to morbid fantasies : sometimes she sees herself pregnant, with everyone staring at her strangely ; one minute she thinks she is a lesbian, the next, a prostitute. She is torn by a conflict which she cannot resolve. As she is too dependent on her parents' approval (they are strait-laced on the subject of contraception), and fears loss of their love if she uses a contraceptive, she seeks refuge in il'ness. Unconsciously she is punishing herself for having violated their moral code.

Some women complain that "it isn't very romantic" to interrupt the flow of love-making in order to prepare for intercourse. Why not take the pill, in that case ? Or have a gynecologist insert an IUD ?

"I often prepare myself before my husband gets home from work," say others ; "I've been disappointed many times when he showed no interest."

"If I were ready all the time, I'd feel like some subject that could be taken or left, depending on how my husband felt," say some.

"The man has all the fun ; why shouldn't he take all the responsibility," I have heard wives say.

Such arguments leave no doubt about these women's true feelings. They resent the "male privilege," rejecting their own feminine role. Very often the husband himself is the object of resentment. In reality, such a woman does not love her husband, either because he does not take care of her as her parents did, or refuses to alter his ideas and opinions as she would like him to. She does not share his interest in sex. She won't refuse his advances, but forgets to prepare herself with a contraceptive, pretends not to be able to find it, or some other more or less plausible excuse. Usually the husband does not have a condom available at the precise moment his wife agrees to use a contraceptive. He puts off the gratification of his sexual urge, or depends on a less reliable method. In this way, the contraceptive becomes a weapon to satisfy the vengeance and hostility which the wife feels towards her husband.

One woman didn't enjoy intercourse because she found the sensation unpleasant. She always had an excuse. Finally, however, the husband had had enough, and didn't care whether she became pregnant or not. He was revenging himself for her lack of interest, and no longer bothered about the question of contraception.

Another woman burst into a storm of tears and complaints in my office, and talked of divorce. "Why all the fuss?" I asked her. Had she not got what she wanted? Probably. Psychiatric examination revealed her desire to be taken by force. She refused to accept this interpretation of her case, but after some thought admitted that following a so-called "rape" she had experienced orgasm for the first time. She was so inhibited that she could not have a complete sexual relation without being forced to do so. Even if she did want intercourse, any erotic foreplay froze her emotionally. Use of a contraceptive went against her conscience, as it amounted to complicity in the forbidden sex act.

There are women who find it uncomfortable or even disgusting to use a diaphragm, which they are obliged to insert in the vagina. This is often linked with parental punishment of masturbation or some other sexual gratification. The hormone pill or IUD, if they are medically suitable, will partially eliminate such resistance. If it is caused by an unconscious fear of sex, however, only a basic change in personality can solve the problem.

Whatever the method of contraception used, its effectiveness depends entirely on the woman and whether she really wishes it to work. Unwanted pregnancies are caused by the woman herself, not by the contraceptive.

Chapter 17
A Final Word

Birth control or contraception is a controversial subject the world over. Surgical sterilization is becoming increasingly widespread. There is a definite trend towards both vasectomy (male surgical sterilization) and salpingectomy (female surgical sterilization), both being permanent forms of contraception — with rare exceptions.

Contraceptive Methods

No method is one hundred per cent foolproof, or without possible side-effects, whether used by the man or the woman : condom or coitus interruptus for the man ; diaphragm, spermicidal creams, the IUD, or contraceptive hormone pill for the woman.

It should be realized that female surgical sterilization, while it offers a permanent method of contraception, causes greater shock to the system than the analogous male operation. It is also more complicated than vasectomy.

A Simple, Effective Operation

Male sterilization does not lead to complications, whereas severing the Fallopian tubes requires an abdominal incision (laparotomy) which is more difficult, longer, more dangerous, and involves a higher stress factor.

For the married couple who are seriously considering permanent contraception, vasectomy is obviously the ideal surgical procedure.

Vasectomy does not alter the composition, volume or appearance of the ejaculation, except that sperm cells are absent. It does not lessen hormone secretion by the testicles, the purpose of which is to stimulate and maintain development of the sexual organs. It does not affect the genital nervous system or a man's physical capacity.

Psychological Effects

Sometimes there is behavioural change. This depends on the man's personality, maturity, the quality of his marital relations, family stability and environment. Because general information about vasectomy in now more widespread, I believe that most men suffer no side-effects of psychological origin, either as to sexual interest or intensity of orgasm. Things remain as they were. I should add that many couples feel that they achieve greater fulfilment in sex. The fear of pregnancy is completely eliminated.

Vasectomy is Not New

The first vasectomy was carried out seventy years ago in the United States by the medical director of a home for mentally retarded teenage boys, in the hope of reducing the incidence of masturbation. The most marked post-operative change which he noticed was sterility.

With the passing years, several American states have legalized sterilization for men and women suffering from mental retardation, epilepsy or mental illness. Only a few permit sterilization of normal individuals, subject to approval by two physicians. If a married couple is involved, the wife's signature is required. In the case of an adolescent, a court decision is required.

Present Opinion

According to American legal experts, men and women have the right to request sterilization for purposes of birth control. The doctor does not act contrary to the law when he proceeds with the permission of the patient and his or her marriage partner.

Vasectomy as a means of contraception is accepted in almost all the over-populated nations. It is basic to the well-being of these nations that their populations be limited. In India, for example, an estimated quarter of a million vasectomies have been performed over the past fifteen years. In the United States, a reputable study carried out by a university group concluded that there were about 45,000 vasectomies carried out annually for contraceptive purposes only. This proves that the trend is toward male sterilization.

I do not see why there is any hesitation about adopting a similar attitude toward contraceptive sterilization — especially vasectomy — in Canada. Vasectomy is simple, totally effective, and not subject to complications. If the husband, wife, and doctor (or two doctors) agree, what could be simpler ? There is nothing dishonest or harmful to anyone involved.

In my view, the important thing is to keep in mind the well-being and capacity for greater fulfilment of both the individual and the family.